I0791785

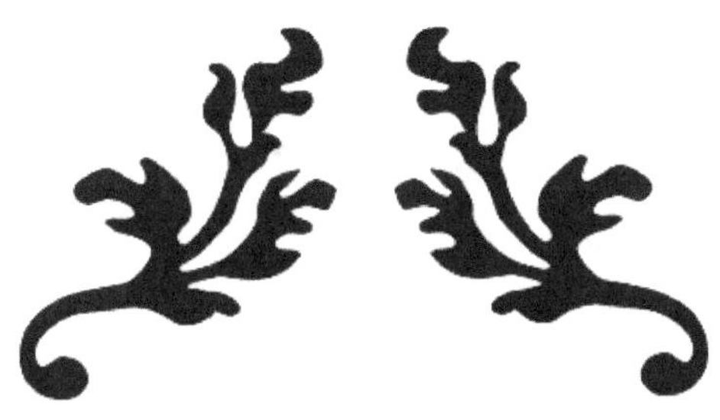

The Castor Oil Bible

A Trusted Guide to Natural Beauty and Everyday Wellness. Effective, Step-by-Step Remedies for Radiant Skin, Healthier Hair, and Whole-Body Relief—Without Any Harsh Chemicals

---

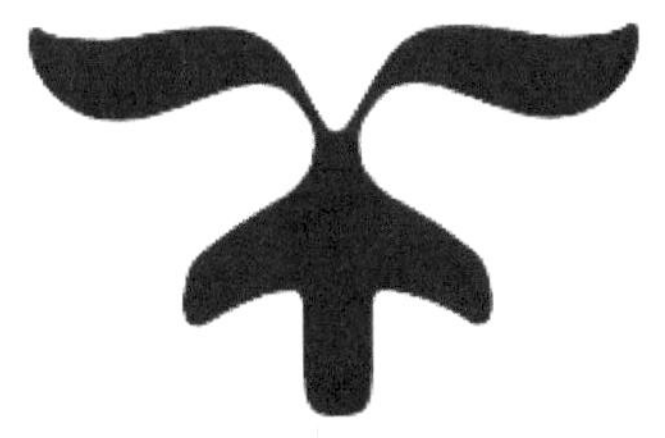

ADA BENNETT

Your journey of transformation starts here…

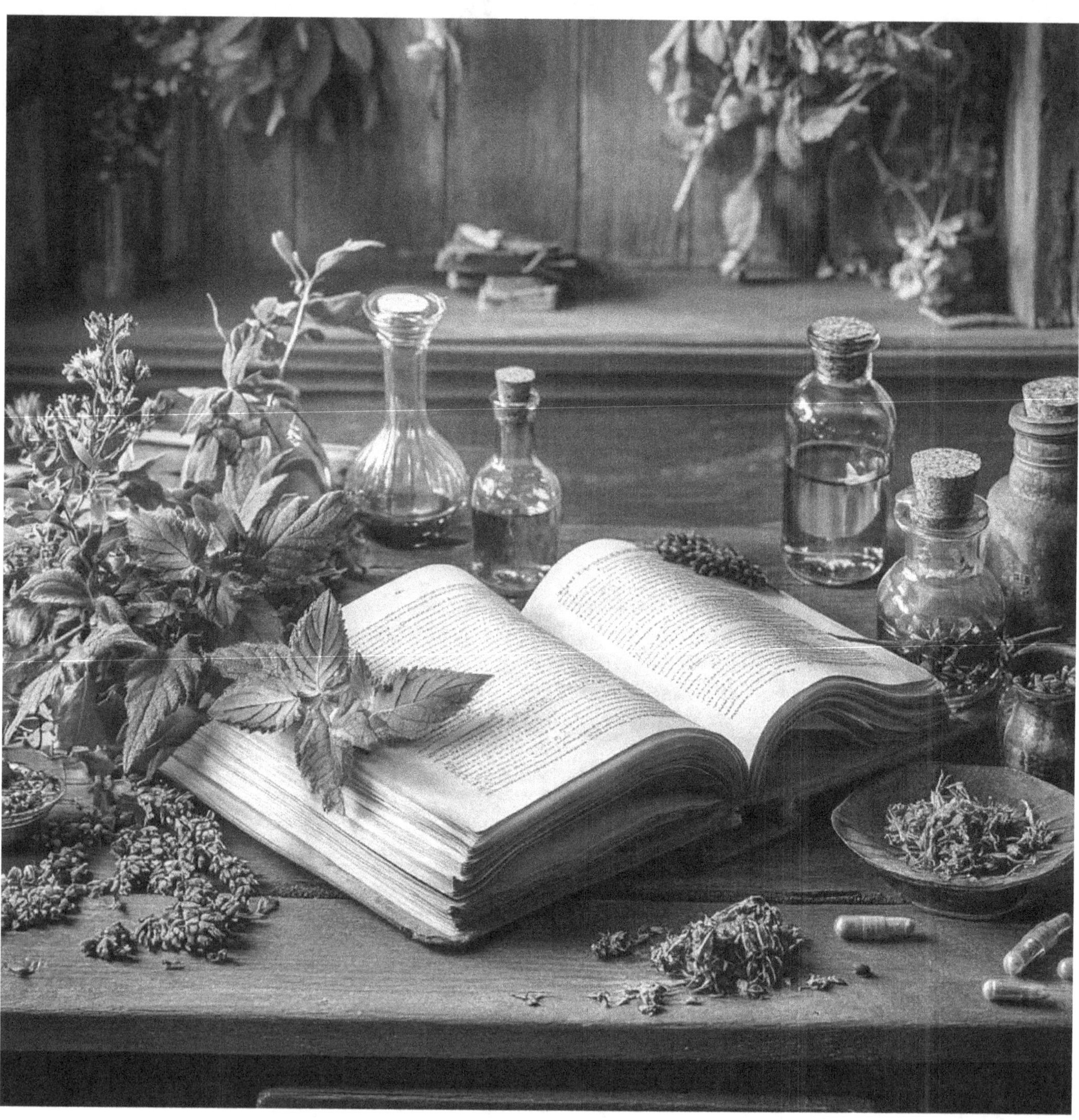

© Copyright 2024 Ada Bennett and Vitalityhealthyvibes all rights reserved.

This document is geared towards providing exact and reliable information with regard to the topic and issue covered. The publication is sold with the idea that the publisher is not required to render accounting, officially permitted, or otherwise qualified services. If advice is necessary, legal or professional, a practiced individual in the profession should be ordered.

From a Declaration of Principles which was accepted and approved equally by a Committee of the American Bar Association and a Committee of Publishers and Associations.

In no way is it legal to reproduce, duplicate, or transmit any part of this document in either electronic means or in printed format. Recording of this publication is strictly prohibited, and any storage of this document is not allowed unless with written permission from the publisher. All rights reserved.

The information provided herein is stated to be truthful and consistent, in that any liability, in terms of inattention or otherwise, by any usage or abuse of any policies, processes, or directions contained within is the solitary and utter responsibility of the recipient reader. Under no circumstances will any legal responsibility or blame be held against the publisher for any reparation, damages, or monetary loss due to the information herein, either directly or indirectly.

Legal Notice:

This book is copyright protected. This book is only for personal use. You cannot amend, distribute, sell, use, quote or paraphrase any part, or the content within this book, without the consent of the author or publisher.

Disclaimer Notice:

This book provides general information. Please note the information contained within this document is for educational and entertainment purposes only. All effort has been executed to present accurate, up to date, and reliable, complete information. No warranties of any kind are declared or implied. Readers acknowledge that the author is not engaging in the rendering of legal, financial, medical or professional advice. The content within this book has been derived from various sources. Please consult a licensed professional before attempting any techniques outlined in this book.

By reading this document, the reader agrees that under no circumstances is the author responsible for any losses, direct or indirect, which are incurred as a result of the use of information contained within this document, including, but not limited to, — errors, omissions, or inaccuracies.

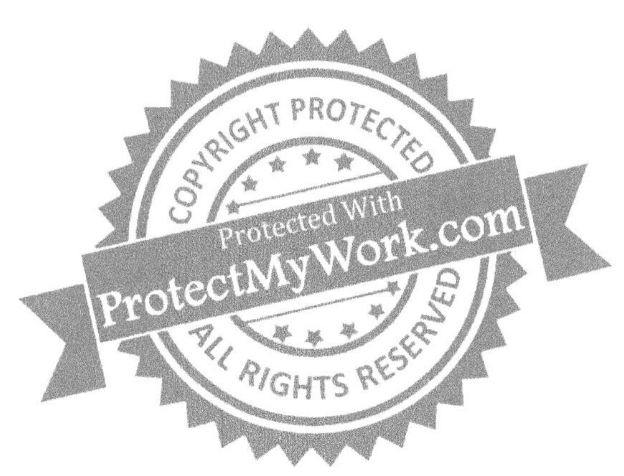

Table of Contents

Introduction to the Power of Castor Oil

The Miracle Oil: What Makes Castor Oil Unique

Imagine a single, natural oil that can nourish your skin, stimulate hair growth, ease discomfort, and support wellness—all without the use of harsh chemicals. Castor oil, often called a "miracle oil," brings together a unique blend of benefits and nutrients, setting it apart as a trusted ally in natural beauty and health.

What makes castor oil so extraordinary is its rich composition. This unassuming oil contains a high concentration of **ricinoleic acid**, a rare fatty acid known for its anti-inflammatory and antimicrobial properties. Ricinoleic acid helps soothe irritated skin, relieve joint and muscle discomfort, and promote overall healing. Additionally, **vitamin E** in castor oil acts as a powerful antioxidant, fighting off free radicals to reduce signs of aging and support cell regeneration. These components work together to create a versatile, nourishing oil suitable for various wellness needs.

Unlike many conventional products filled with synthetic additives, castor oil stands out for its simplicity and purity. By incorporating castor oil into your routine, you're embracing a solution that's both effective and rooted in nature, offering a gentle approach that aligns with the body's natural processes. As you explore the pages ahead, you'll discover how this time-tested oil can bring balance, radiance, and comfort to your daily life. Castor oil is not just an ordinary remedy; it's a safe, natural, and accessible way to enhance your well-being in multiple dimensions.

Castor Oil Through History: Ancient to Modern Uses

Castor oil's reputation as a healing, beautifying oil has been cultivated over thousands of years, crossing cultures and continents. From the **ancient Egyptians**, who used castor oil for skin care and as a powerful healing agent, to **traditional Ayurvedic practitioners in India**, who employed it for detoxification and balancing the body's energies, castor oil has long been treasured as a potent natural remedy.

In ancient Greece, it was recognized as a valuable aid for soothing the body and enhancing beauty. Castor oil was even found in Egyptian tombs, symbolizing its revered status in wellness and beauty routines of the past. Fast-forward to today, and castor oil's uses have only expanded, now encompassing remedies for skin hydration, hair growth, pain relief, and more.

By choosing to incorporate castor oil into your life, you're not only tapping into a time-honored tradition but also embracing a modern approach to wellness that values simplicity, purity, and natural effectiveness. This blend of ancient wisdom and contemporary knowledge positions castor oil as an enduring, reliable choice for anyone seeking gentle yet impactful results.

How to Use This Book for Health, Beauty, and Wellness

This book is your personal guide to unlocking the transformative benefits of castor oil in ways that align with your health, beauty, and wellness goals. Each chapter provides straightforward, step-by-step insights into specific uses for castor oil, whether you're looking to nurture your skin, enhance hair health, relieve discomfort, or simply integrate more natural remedies into your daily routine.

Designed with both beginners and experienced users in mind, each section offers accessible guidance, empowering you to take actionable steps with confidence. You'll find practical applications, DIY recipes, and tips that make incorporating castor oil into your life both simple and rewarding. Whether your aim is to rejuvenate your skin, promote relaxation, or support overall well-being, each page is crafted to provide clear, achievable steps to help you on your journey.

This book isn't just a compilation of recipes and remedies; it's an invitation to explore the full potential of castor oil, transforming your approach to self-care and natural wellness. Dive in and discover how this remarkable oil can be a valuable, easy-to-use ally in your pursuit of a balanced, radiant, and healthful life.

The Science Behind Castor Oil

Key Components: Ricinoleic Acid and Other Compounds

At the heart of castor oil's remarkable benefits lies its unique chemical makeup, especially its high concentration of **ricinoleic acid**. This powerful fatty acid is rarely found in other oils, making castor oil stand out as a potent natural remedy. Ricinoleic acid is known for its **anti-inflammatory and antimicrobial properties**, helping soothe irritated skin, reduce joint pain, and promote healing in a natural, gentle way.

Beyond ricinoleic acid, castor oil contains a variety of beneficial nutrients, including **vitamin E**—an antioxidant that combats skin damage and aging. Its **omega fatty acids** help nourish and moisturize, providing deep hydration that supports skin elasticity and softness. Castor oil also holds antioxidants that protect cells from oxidative stress, promoting overall skin health and radiance. These components work together to create an oil that is both versatile and deeply nourishing, making it ideal for a wide range of beauty and wellness applications.

In simpler terms, think of castor oil as a nutrient-rich elixir that naturally targets common concerns like dryness, inflammation, and discomfort. It's a blend of nature's finest ingredients that doesn't require additives to deliver real, noticeable benefits.

How Castor Oil Works: Healing, Inflammation Reduction, and Detox

So, how exactly does castor oil work its magic? One of its main effects is **reducing inflammation**, thanks to the unique properties of ricinoleic acid. When applied to the skin or used in castor oil packs, it penetrates deeply, helping to soothe sore muscles, ease joint pain, and calm irritated skin. Its anti-inflammatory effects make it a popular choice for individuals dealing with discomfort from arthritis, mild skin rashes, or muscle tension after a long day.

Another fascinating aspect of castor oil is its ability to support the body's **detox and immune functions**. When used in castor oil packs, it encourages **lymphatic drainage**, helping the body to remove toxins more efficiently and boosting circulation. By improving blood flow and aiding the lymphatic system, castor oil enhances the body's natural detox processes, promoting a sense of renewal and well-being.

Think of castor oil as a nutrient delivery system: it reaches deep into the skin to provide targeted relief and support the body's natural functions. This unique ability to penetrate layers of tissue means that castor oil doesn't just sit on the surface; it works within, offering a depth of care that's hard to find in other natural oils.

Scientific Studies and Research-Backed Benefits

While castor oil has centuries of traditional use behind it, modern science also backs many of its benefits. Numerous studies have highlighted castor oil's **moisturizing properties** for skin. Research shows that it can significantly increase skin hydration, making it a reliable remedy for those with dry, cracked, or aging skin.

Hair growth is another area where castor oil has demonstrated real promise. Studies indicate that its ability to stimulate circulation and nourish hair follicles can support thicker, healthier hair over time. Additionally, research on castor oil's anti-inflammatory effects supports its use for **pain relief**, especially in cases of mild arthritis or muscle soreness.

These findings underscore castor oil's potential as a scientifically supported natural remedy—not just a folk solution passed down through generations. Knowing that castor oil is backed by reliable research should reassure readers that they're making a safe, informed choice in using it for their wellness needs.

Debunking Myths and Misconceptions

Despite its many benefits, castor oil has sometimes been surrounded by myths or misconceptions. One common myth is that **castor oil is toxic**—a misconception that likely arises from the fact that castor seeds, if ingested whole, contain ricin, a harmful substance. However, the oil itself is entirely safe for topical use and can even be taken internally in small, carefully regulated doses.

Another misconception is that castor oil can work as a "miracle cure" for all health issues. While it offers numerous benefits, it's essential to understand that castor oil is a supportive remedy rather than an instant fix. Its effects are best appreciated over time and through consistent use.

These clarifications help separate fact from fiction, allowing readers to move forward with confidence. When used properly, castor oil is a safe, effective, and versatile addition to a natural wellness routine.

Properties, Selection, and Storage of Castor Oil

Types of Castor Oil: Organic, Cold-Pressed, and Refined

Castor oil comes in several forms, each with unique benefits tailored to different uses. Understanding these types can help you choose the best option for your needs, whether you're focusing on skin care, hair health, or wellness routines.

1. **Organic Castor Oil**: This type of castor oil is derived from castor beans grown without the use of synthetic pesticides or fertilizers, making it a cleaner, more natural option. Organic castor oil is ideal for those who prioritize purity and prefer a product with minimal processing. This type is especially popular for beauty and wellness applications, where high-quality, toxin-free ingredients are essential.
2. **Cold-Pressed Castor Oil**: Extracted without heat, cold-pressed castor oil retains a higher concentration of nutrients, including essential fatty acids and antioxidants. This gentle extraction method helps maintain the oil's natural effectiveness, making cold-pressed oil a top choice for skin and hair care. If you're looking for a product that offers maximum moisturizing and healing properties, cold-pressed is an excellent option.
3. **Refined Castor Oil**: Unlike organic or cold-pressed varieties, refined castor oil undergoes additional processing to remove impurities and odors, often resulting in a lighter color and milder scent. While it may lack some of the nutrients found in cold-pressed oil, refined castor oil is still useful for applications where purity isn't as critical, such as in industrial uses or DIY crafts.

Each type of castor oil offers unique benefits, so selecting the right one depends on how you plan to use it. For beauty and health applications, organic and cold-pressed oils are generally preferred for their nutrient density and purity, while refined options work well for more general or household uses.

How to Select and Purchase High-Quality Castor Oil

With so many brands and types of castor oil on the market, finding a high-quality option can feel overwhelming. Here are some tips to guide you in choosing a safe, effective product:

- **Look for Labels like "Organic" and "Cold-Pressed"**: Organic labels ensure that the oil is free from pesticides, while cold-pressed labels indicate a gentle extraction process that preserves the oil's natural nutrients.
- **Check for Certifications**: Certifications like USDA Organic can help you identify products that meet rigorous quality standards. These certifications confirm that the castor oil has been produced with minimal environmental impact and is free from synthetic additives.
- **Read the Ingredient List Carefully**: Quality castor oil should be pure and free from additives or fillers. Look for labels that list "100% castor oil" as the only ingredient, as added chemicals can reduce the effectiveness of the oil, especially for beauty or wellness applications.

- **Choose Reputable Brands**: Established brands often provide better transparency regarding sourcing and processing methods. Look for brands with good customer reviews and a reputation for quality to avoid lower-quality options.

By taking these steps, you can ensure that the castor oil you choose is pure, effective, and safe for use in your health and beauty routines.

Proper Storage for Maximum Freshness and Potency

To get the most out of your castor oil, proper storage is essential. Following these simple guidelines can help you maintain the oil's quality and effectiveness over time:

- **Store in a Cool, Dark Place**: Exposure to heat and sunlight can degrade castor oil, reducing its potency and shelf life. Keep the oil in a cool, shaded area, such as a cupboard, away from direct sunlight and heat sources.
- **Use an Airtight Container**: Exposure to air can accelerate the breakdown of castor oil, so make sure it's stored in a tightly sealed container. Glass containers are ideal, as they don't react with the oil, but if the product comes in plastic packaging, ensure it's food-grade and BPA-free.
- **Check for Signs of Expiration**: While castor oil generally has a long shelf life, it's still important to check for any signs of spoilage, such as a rancid smell or unusual cloudiness. Properly stored, castor oil can last up to a year, but if it starts to smell off, it's best to replace it.

By following these steps, you can keep your castor oil fresh and effective, ensuring that it provides all the intended benefits without degradation over time.

Essential Safety Tips for Using Castor Oil

Castor oil is generally safe for a wide range of applications, but a few simple precautions can help ensure optimal results and prevent any adverse effects:

- **Do a Patch Test First**: Before applying castor oil to larger areas of skin, test a small amount on your wrist or inner arm to check for any sensitivities. This step is especially important for those with sensitive skin or a history of allergies.
- **Follow Dosage Guidelines for Internal Use**: If you're considering internal use of castor oil, consult a healthcare provider for guidance on safe dosage, as even natural remedies can have side effects if overused. Generally, only small, regulated amounts are recommended for laxative purposes, and long-term internal use should be avoided unless directed by a professional.
- **Use with Caution Around Eyes and Mucous Membranes**: While castor oil is often used safely for eyelashes and brows, avoid getting it directly into your eyes or other sensitive areas. If applying around the eye area, use only a tiny amount and proceed with care.
- **Keep Out of Reach of Children**: Though castor oil is natural, it's important to store it safely, especially if children are in the home. Some children may be sensitive to the oil, and ingestion in large quantities can cause discomfort.

When used with care, castor oil is a safe, effective addition to your natural wellness routine. By following these basic safety tips, you can confidently enjoy the numerous benefits it offers.

Skin Care and Beauty with Castor Oil

Moisturization and Hydration: For Dry Skin, Rough Patches, and Cracked Heels

Castor oil's deeply moisturizing properties make it a powerful remedy for dry skin, rough patches, and cracked heels. Thanks to its rich concentration of fatty acids, castor oil penetrates deeply into the skin, providing lasting hydration and nourishment. It's especially effective for areas that are prone to dryness, like hands, elbows, and feet, leaving skin soft and smooth with regular use.

Application Tips:

- Apply a few drops of castor oil directly to damp skin after a shower to lock in moisture.
- For rough patches or cracked heels, gently massage a small amount into the area before bed and wear cotton gloves or socks to help the oil absorb overnight.
- Consider blending castor oil with lighter oils, like coconut or almond oil, for a hydrating mix that's easy to apply.

Deep Moisture Hand Balm

Purpose/Benefits: Provides long-lasting hydration and repair for dry, cracked hands.

Ingredients:

- 1 tablespoon castor oil (organic, cold-pressed)
- 1 tablespoon shea butter
- 1 teaspoon beeswax
- 3 drops lavender essential oil (optional)

Tools/Equipment:

- Small saucepan
- Mixing spoon
- Small container with lid

Instructions:

1. Melt the beeswax and shea butter in a small saucepan over low heat.
2. Remove from heat and stir in the castor oil and lavender essential oil.
3. Pour the mixture into a container and allow it to cool and solidify.

Application Tips:

- Apply to hands as needed, especially after washing or exposure to cold.

Storage and Shelf Life:

- Store in a cool, dry place. Shelf life is approximately 6 months.

Safety Notes:

- For external use only. Perform a patch test before full application.

Hydrating Body Scrub with Castor Oil and Sugar

Purpose/Benefits: Exfoliates and deeply moisturizes, leaving skin soft and smooth.

Ingredients:

- 1 tablespoon castor oil
- 1 tablespoon coconut oil
- 2 tablespoons fine sugar
- 1 drop peppermint essential oil (optional)

Tools/Equipment:

- Small bowl

Instructions:

1. Combine castor oil, coconut oil, and sugar.
2. Add peppermint oil if desired and mix thoroughly.

Application Tips:

- Gently massage onto damp skin in circular motions, then rinse.

Storage and Shelf Life:

- Prepare fresh for each use.

Calming Facial Mist with Castor Oil and Rose Water

Purpose/Benefits: Refreshes and hydrates skin throughout the day.

Ingredients:

- ½ teaspoon castor oil
- 1 cup rose water
- 3 drops chamomile essential oil (optional)

Tools/Equipment:

- Small spray bottle

Instructions:

1. Add all ingredients to the spray bottle.
2. Shake well before each use.

Application Tips:

- Mist over the face as needed to hydrate and calm skin.

Storage and Shelf Life:

- Store in a cool, dry place. Shelf life is 2 weeks.

Safety Notes:

- Shake well to disperse oils before spraying on the face.

Castor Oil Hand and Nail Balm for Rough, Dry Hands

Purpose/Benefits: Moisturizes dry hands and strengthens nails.

Ingredients:

- 1 tablespoon castor oil
- 1 tablespoon shea butter
- 1 teaspoon olive oil

Tools/Equipment:

- Mixing bowl
- Small container

Instructions:

1. Blend castor oil, shea butter, and olive oil in a bowl until smooth.
2. Transfer to a container.

Application Tips:

- Apply to hands and nails as needed, especially before bed.

Storage and Shelf Life:

- Store at room temperature; lasts up to 3 months.

Safety Notes:

- Keep away from eyes.

Anti-Aging Properties: Reducing Wrinkles, Fine Lines, and Free Radical Damage

Castor oil is a natural powerhouse when it comes to fighting the signs of aging. Its antioxidant properties help combat free radicals, one of the main contributors to wrinkles and fine lines. Additionally, castor oil supports skin elasticity, making it a valuable ally in maintaining a youthful glow without resorting to conventional, chemical-laden anti-aging products.

How to Use for Anti-Aging:

- Gently massage a few drops of castor oil onto your face and neck in upward circular motions, focusing on areas with fine lines. Doing this at night allows the oil to nourish your skin as you sleep.
- For added anti-aging benefits, combine castor oil with essential oils known for skin rejuvenation, such as frankincense or rosehip oil. Just a few drops of each can enhance castor oil's effects.

Rejuvenating Anti-Aging Face Serum

Purpose/Benefits: Helps reduce the appearance of fine lines and promotes youthful skin.

Ingredients:

- 1 teaspoon castor oil (organic, cold-pressed)
- 1 teaspoon argan oil
- 3 drops frankincense essential oil

Tools/Equipment:

- Small dropper bottle

Instructions:

1. Combine castor oil, argan oil, and frankincense oil in the dropper bottle.
2. Shake gently to mix.

Application Tips:

- Apply a few drops to clean skin at night, focusing on areas prone to fine lines.

Storage and Shelf Life:

- Store in a cool, dark place. Shelf life is 6 months.

Safety Notes:

- Avoid the eye area and perform a patch test before use.

Anti-Aging Face Serum for Men

Purpose/Benefits: Reduces the appearance of fine lines and hydrates skin.

Ingredients:

- 1 tablespoon castor oil
- 1 teaspoon vitamin E oil
- 2 drops frankincense essential oil

Tools/Equipment:

- Dropper bottle

Instructions:

1. Mix all oils in the dropper bottle.

Application Tips:

- Apply a few drops to clean skin at night for best results.

Storage and Shelf Life:

- Store in a cool, dark place; lasts up to 6 months.

Safety Notes:

- Patch test before using to ensure no sensitivity.

Firming Neck and Décolletage Cream

Purpose/Benefits: Tightens and nourishes delicate neck and chest skin.

Ingredients:

- 1 tablespoon castor oil
- 1 teaspoon rosehip oil
- 2 drops geranium essential oil

Tools/Equipment:

- Small container

Instructions:

1. Combine all ingredients in a container and mix well.

Application Tips:

- Apply to the neck and décolletage nightly.

Storage and Shelf Life:

- Store in a cool, dark place. Shelf life is 6 months.

Soothing Castor Oil Under-Eye Cream for Tired Eyes

Purpose/Benefits: Reduces puffiness and dark circles.

Ingredients:

- 1 teaspoon castor oil
- 1 teaspoon aloe vera gel
- 2 drops cucumber extract (optional)

Tools/Equipment:

- Small container

Instructions:

1. Mix all ingredients in the container until well-blended.

Application Tips:

- Dab a small amount under each eye at night.

Storage and Shelf Life:

- Store in the fridge; lasts up to 2 weeks.

Safety Notes:

- Avoid direct contact with the eyes.

Acne Treatment: Combating Inflammation and Bacterial Buildup

For those with acne-prone skin, castor oil's antibacterial and anti-inflammatory properties offer a gentle, natural solution. Its main compound, ricinoleic acid, helps reduce inflammation and controls bacterial growth, addressing two primary causes of acne. Unlike some harsher treatments, castor oil soothes rather than irritates, making it a beneficial addition to an acne-care routine.

Application Methods:

- For spot treatment, apply a small amount of castor oil to blemishes using a cotton swab, leaving it on overnight before rinsing in the morning.
- If you prefer a lighter application, blend castor oil with jojoba oil, which helps balance sebum production, for an effective, all-over facial oil.

Clear Complexion Acne Spot Treatment

Purpose/Benefits: Targets acne by reducing inflammation and combating bacteria.

Ingredients:

- ½ teaspoon castor oil
- 1 drop tea tree essential oil

Tools/Equipment:

- Small bowl
- Cotton swab

Instructions:

1. Mix castor oil and tea tree oil in a small bowl.
2. Apply a small amount to blemishes using a cotton swab.

Application Tips:

- Use as a spot treatment once a day until the blemish clears.

Storage and Shelf Life:

- Prepare fresh for each use.

Safety Notes:

- Avoid large areas of skin as tea tree oil can be drying.

Blackhead Dissolving Pore Cleanser

Purpose/Benefits: Reduces blackheads and helps refine pores with a gentle, natural formula.

Ingredients:

- 1 teaspoon castor oil
- 1 teaspoon jojoba oil
- 1 teaspoon honey

Tools/Equipment:

- Small bowl
- Cotton pads (optional)

Instructions:

1. Mix castor oil, jojoba oil, and honey in a small bowl.
2. Apply to clean skin, focusing on blackhead-prone areas.

Application Tips:

- Massage gently for 1-2 minutes, then rinse with warm water.
- Use 1-2 times a week.

Storage and Shelf Life:

- Prepare fresh for each use.
- Avoid applying to broken or irritated skin.

Safety Notes:

Eczema and Psoriasis Relief: Soothing Itching, Irritation, and Inflammation

Castor oil is renowned for its soothing properties, making it a comforting option for those struggling with eczema or psoriasis. Its rich, hydrating quality helps to calm itching and irritation, while its anti-inflammatory effects reduce redness and inflammation associated with these skin conditions.

Application Suggestions:

- For flare-ups, create a soothing balm by combining castor oil with coconut oil or shea butter. Apply it to affected areas for immediate relief.
- Another option is to apply a few drops of castor oil directly to irritated skin, massaging gently to avoid further irritation.

Gentle Eczema Relief Cream

Purpose/Benefits: Soothes and calms irritated skin, relieving eczema symptoms.

Ingredients:

- 1 tablespoon castor oil
- 1 tablespoon coconut oil
- 1 drop chamomile essential oil (optional)

Tools/Equipment:

- Small container with lid

Instructions:

1. Combine castor oil, coconut oil, and chamomile oil in the container.
2. Mix until well blended.

Application Tips:

- Apply to affected areas as needed.

Storage and Shelf Life:

- Store in a cool, dry place. Shelf life is 3 months.

Safety Notes:

- Perform a patch test to ensure no irritation occurs.

<u>**Psoriasis Soothing Body Oil**</u>

Purpose/Benefits: Calms inflammation and relieves itchiness associated with psoriasis.

Ingredients:

- 1 tablespoon castor oil
- 1 tablespoon jojoba oil
- 2 drops tea tree essential oil

Tools/Equipment:

- Small container

Instructions:

1. Combine all oils in a container and mix well.

Application Tips:

- Apply to affected areas as needed.

Storage and Shelf Life:

- Shelf life is 3 months.

Lip Care and Healing Balms: Hydrating and Repairing Cracked or Chapped Lips

Castor oil's rich, hydrating properties also make it an excellent choice for lip care. It provides long-lasting moisture, ideal for repairing dry, cracked lips, and can be combined with other nourishing ingredients to create a simple, effective DIY lip balm.

<u>**Healing Lip Repair Balm**</u>

Purpose/Benefits: Restores moisture and smoothness to chapped lips.

Ingredients:

- 1 teaspoon castor oil
- 1 teaspoon beeswax
- ½ teaspoon coconut oil

Tools/Equipment:

- Small saucepan
- Lip balm container

Instructions:

1. Melt beeswax and coconut oil in a saucepan.
2. Add castor oil and stir.
3. Pour into a container and let it solidify.

Application Tips:

- Apply to lips as needed.

Storage and Shelf Life:

- Shelf life is 6 months

Natural Sunscreen Balm with Castor Oil

Purpose/Benefits: Provides daily UV protection without chemicals.

Ingredients:

- 1 tablespoon castor oil
- 1 tablespoon coconut oil
- 1 tablespoon zinc oxide powder

Tools/Equipment:

- Mixing bowl
- Small container

Instructions:

1. Combine castor oil, coconut oil, and zinc oxide in a bowl until smooth.
2. Transfer to a container.

Application Tips:

- Apply to skin before sun exposure.

Storage and Shelf Life:

- Store at room temperature; lasts up to 3 months.

Safety Notes:

- Not suitable for prolonged sun exposure or water activities.

DIY Foot Balm with Castor Oil for Calluses and Dryness

Purpose/Benefits: Softens calluses and deeply moisturizes dry feet.

Ingredients:

- 1 tablespoon castor oil
- 1 tablespoon cocoa butter
- 2 drops peppermint essential oil

Tools/Equipment:

- Mixing bowl
- Storage container

Instructions:

1. Melt the cocoa butter, then add castor oil and peppermint oil.
2. Stir until smooth and pour into the container.

Application Tips:

- Apply to feet at night and wear socks for better absorption.

Storage and Shelf Life:

- Store in a cool place; lasts up to 3 months.

Safety Notes:

- Avoid contact with open wounds.

Brightening Eye and Under-Eye Treatment

Find natural solutions for dark circles and puffiness with castor oil, which brightens and refreshes delicate under-eye skin.

Brightening Under-Eye Serum

Purpose/Benefits: Reduces dark circles and puffiness, giving a refreshed look.

Ingredients:

- ½ teaspoon castor oil
- ½ teaspoon sweet almond oil
- 1 drop vitamin E oil (optional)

Tools/Equipment:

- Small bottle with roller or dropper

Instructions:

1. Combine castor oil, almond oil, and vitamin E oil in a bottle.
2. Shake well.

Application Tips:

- Apply a small amount around the under-eye area at night.

Storage and Shelf Life:

- Store in a cool, dark place. Shelf life is 3 months.

DIY Recipes for Radiant Skin: Hydrating Masks, Anti-Aging Serums, and Balms

Castor oil can be used in various DIY recipes that offer targeted benefits for different skincare needs. Here are a few beginner-friendly recipes to help you create radiant, healthy skin:

Nourishing Overnight Face Mask

Purpose/Benefits: Deeply hydrates and revitalizes skin overnight.

Ingredients:

- 1 tablespoon castor oil
- 1 tablespoon aloe vera gel
- 2 drops lavender essential oil

Tools/Equipment:

- Small bowl

- Application brush (optional)

Instructions:

1. Mix castor oil, aloe vera gel, and lavender oil.
2. Apply a thin layer to clean skin before bed.

Application Tips:

- Use 1-2 times a week.

Storage and Shelf Life:

- Prepare fresh for each use.

Sunburn Relief Gel with Castor Oil and Aloe Vera

Purpose/Benefits: Soothes sunburned skin and reduces inflammation.

Ingredients:

- 1 tablespoon castor oil
- 2 tablespoons aloe vera gel
- 3 drops lavender essential oil (optional)

Tools/Equipment:

- Small bowl
- Spoon for mixing

Instructions:

1. Combine castor oil and aloe vera gel in the bowl.
2. Add lavender oil if desired and mix well.

Application Tips:

- Apply a thin layer to sunburned areas as needed for relief.

Storage and Shelf Life:

- Store in a cool, dark place. Use within 1 week for best results.

Safety Notes:

- Avoid applying to broken or severely blistered skin.

Skin Brightening Face Toner

Purpose/Benefits: A natural toner that evens out skin tone and adds radiance.

Ingredients:

- 1 teaspoon castor oil
- 1 cup rose water
- 1 teaspoon apple cider vinegar

Tools/Equipment:

- Spray bottle or small bottle with lid

Instructions:

1. Mix castor oil, rose water, and apple cider vinegar in the bottle.
2. Shake well before each use.

Application Tips:

- After cleansing, apply toner with a cotton pad or spray on the face.

Storage and Shelf Life:

- Store in a cool, dry place. Shelf life is 1 month.

Safety Notes:

- Perform a patch test first as apple cider vinegar can be irritating for sensitive skin.

Stretch Mark & Scar Reduction Oil

Purpose/Benefits: Helps reduce the appearance of scars and stretch marks with consistent use.

Ingredients:

- 1 tablespoon castor oil
- 1 tablespoon rosehip oil
- 5 drops frankincense essential oil

Tools/Equipment:

- Small container

Instructions:

1. Mix castor oil, rosehip oil, and frankincense oil in a container.
2. Stir or shake well to combine.

Application Tips:

- Massage onto affected areas once daily for best results.

Storage and Shelf Life:

- Store in a cool, dark place. Shelf life is 6 months.

Safety Notes:

- Avoid applying to open wounds or fresh scars.

Each recipe provides a simple way to incorporate castor oil into your skincare routine, giving you the freedom to customize your approach based on your skin's needs.

Hair Care and Scalp Health with Castor Oil

Hair Growth Promotion: Stimulating Follicles and Improving Circulation

Castor oil is a trusted choice for promoting hair growth, thanks to its high concentration of ricinoleic acid. This unique compound not only nourishes the scalp but also stimulates blood flow to the hair follicles, creating a healthier environment for hair growth. Consistent use can help support fuller, more resilient hair by delivering essential nutrients directly to the scalp.

Application Tips:

- Massage a small amount of castor oil onto your scalp using gentle, circular motions to encourage circulation. Leave it on for 30 minutes to an hour, then rinse.
- For an extra boost, combine castor oil with a few drops of rosemary or peppermint essential oil. These oils enhance circulation and add an invigorating feel to your scalp massage.

Hair Growth Boosting Scalp Serum

Purpose/Benefits: Encourages hair growth by stimulating the scalp with castor oil and peppermint oil.

Ingredients:

- 1 tablespoon castor oil
- 1 tablespoon jojoba oil
- 5 drops peppermint essential oil

Tools/Equipment:

- Small dropper bottle or container

Instructions:

1. Combine castor oil, jojoba oil, and peppermint oil in the dropper bottle.
2. Shake well to blend the oils.

Application Tips:

- Apply a few drops to the scalp, gently massaging in circular motions. Use 2-3 times a week for best results.

Storage and Shelf Life:

- Store in a cool, dark place. Shelf life is 3 months.

Safety Notes:

- Perform a patch test before full application to check for scalp sensitivity to peppermint oil.

Deep Conditioning Castor Oil Hair Mask

Purpose/Benefits: Nourishes and repairs dry or damaged hair for improved texture and resilience.

Ingredients:

- 2 tablespoons castor oil
- 1 tablespoon coconut oil
- 1 tablespoon honey

Tools/Equipment:

- Small bowl
- Application brush (optional)

Instructions:

1. Combine castor oil, coconut oil, and honey in a bowl, mixing until smooth.
2. Apply to damp hair, focusing on the lengths and ends.

Application Tips:

- Leave on for 30-45 minutes, then wash out with shampoo. Use once a week.

Storage and Shelf Life:

- Prepare fresh each time for maximum effectiveness.

Safety Notes:

- Use a shower cap or towel to cover hair during the mask treatment for easier cleanup.

Castor Oil Scalp Treatment for Itchy Skin

Purpose/Benefits: Relieves dryness and itchiness on the scalp, providing nourishment.

Ingredients:

- 1 tablespoon castor oil
- 1 tablespoon coconut oil
- 5 drops tea tree essential oil

Tools/Equipment:

- Small bowl

Instructions:

1. Combine all ingredients in the bowl.
2. Mix until well blended.

Application Tips:

- Massage into the scalp and leave on for 20 minutes before rinsing with warm water.

Storage and Shelf Life:

- Store in a cool place. Use within 1 week.

Safety Notes:

Perform a patch test to ensure no sensitivity to tea tree oil.

Castor Oil Scalp Massage Oil for Hair Growth and Health

Purpose/Benefits: Stimulates follicles for healthy hair growth through regular scalp massage.

Ingredients:

- 1 tablespoon castor oil
- 1 tablespoon olive oil
- 2 drops rosemary essential oil

Tools/Equipment:

- Small bottle

Instructions:

1. Mix ingredients in the bottle.

Application Tips:

- Massage onto scalp weekly for 5-10 minutes, then rinse.

Storage and Shelf Life:

- Store in a cool place; lasts up to 6 months.

Safety Notes:

- Perform a patch test before full use.

Strengthening Hair and Preventing Breakage: Moisturizing and Strengthening

One of castor oil's standout qualities is its deep moisturizing ability. By sealing moisture into the hair strands, castor oil helps prevent breakage and split ends, making it especially beneficial for dry or brittle hair. Its rich texture provides a protective barrier, adding resilience, shine, and an extra layer of defense against damage.

Methods for Strengthening Hair:

- Apply a few drops of castor oil to the ends of your hair, particularly if they are prone to dryness or split ends. This locks in moisture and adds softness.
- For a nourishing treatment, mix castor oil with coconut oil and apply it from mid-length to the ends of your hair. Leave it on for an hour or overnight before rinsing for a deeply hydrating boost.

Split-End Repair Treatment

Purpose/Benefits: Minimizes split ends and breakage, enhancing hair health and smoothness.

Ingredients:

- 1 tablespoon castor oil
- 1 teaspoon argan oil

Tools/Equipment:

- Small bowl

Instructions:

1. Mix castor oil and argan oil in a bowl.

2. Apply sparingly to the ends of your hair.

Application Tips:

- Use 1-2 times per week, focusing only on split ends.

Storage and Shelf Life:

- Store in a cool place for up to 6 months.

Safety Notes:

- Avoid applying too much to prevent a greasy look.

Anti-Frizz Smoothing Hair Oil

Purpose/Benefits: Controls frizz and adds moisture, especially in humid climates.

Ingredients:

- 1 teaspoon castor oil
- 1 teaspoon almond oil
- 2 drops rosemary essential oil (optional)

Tools/Equipment:

- Small container

Instructions:

1. Combine oils in the container.
2. Apply a small amount to damp or dry hair, focusing on ends.

Application Tips:

- Use sparingly as needed, particularly in humid weather.

Storage and Shelf Life:

- Store for up to 6 months in a cool place.

Safety Notes:

- Patch test for sensitivity to rosemary oil if added.

Hair Thickening Scalp Treatment with Castor Oil

Purpose/Benefits: Supports hair thickness and scalp health.

Ingredients:

- 1 tablespoon castor oil
- 1 tablespoon argan oil
- 3 drops tea tree essential oil

Tools/Equipment:

- Small bottle

Instructions:

1. Combine the oils in a bottle and shake to blend.

Application Tips:

- Massage into the scalp weekly and leave on for 20 minutes before rinsing.

Storage and Shelf Life:

- Store in a cool place; lasts up to 6 months.

Safety Notes:

- Patch test before full application.

Dandruff and Scalp Health: Antifungal and Anti-Inflammatory Properties

If you struggle with dandruff or an itchy, flaky scalp, castor oil's antifungal and anti-inflammatory qualities provide natural relief. It can help combat the underlying causes of dandruff, such as scalp irritation or fungal growth, offering a gentle yet effective alternative to harsher chemical treatments.

Application Ideas:

- Use castor oil alone or mix it with a few drops of tea tree oil for enhanced antifungal effects. Massage into the scalp, focusing on problem areas, and leave on for at least 30 minutes before rinsing.
- For ongoing maintenance, apply a small amount of castor oil to your scalp once or twice weekly to keep itchiness and flakiness at bay.

Anti-Dandruff Scalp Soother

Purpose/Benefits: Reduces dandruff and soothes irritation with castor oil and tea tree oil.

Ingredients:

- 1 tablespoon castor oil
- 1 tablespoon olive oil
- 3 drops tea tree essential oil

Tools/Equipment:

- Small bowl

Instructions:

1. Mix castor oil, olive oil, and tea tree oil in the bowl.
2. Apply directly to the scalp, massaging gently.

Application Tips:

- Leave on for 15-20 minutes, then rinse thoroughly. Use 1-2 times a week.

Storage and Shelf Life:

- Store any leftover oil in a cool, dark place for up to 1 month.

Safety Notes:

- Do a patch test for tea tree oil sensitivity.

Scalp Massage Oil for Circulation and Relaxation

Purpose/Benefits: Boosts circulation and relaxation through scalp massage.

Ingredients:

- 1 tablespoon castor oil
- 1 tablespoon grapeseed oil
- 3 drops lavender essential oil

Tools/Equipment:

- Small container

Instructions:

1. Combine all oils in the container.
2. Massage gently onto the scalp for 5-10 minutes.

Application Tips:

- Use once a week as a relaxing scalp massage treatment.

Storage and Shelf Life:

- Store in a cool, dark place. Shelf life is 3 months.

Safety Notes:

- Avoid direct eye contact with oils.

Eyelash and Eyebrow Care: Thicken and Condition Lashes and Brows

Castor oil is a simple, effective way to promote thicker, healthier eyelashes and eyebrows. Its conditioning properties nourish delicate hair follicles, encouraging fuller growth over time. When applied sparingly, castor oil helps create strong, defined lashes and brows without needing chemical-based enhancers.

Simple Lash and Brow Treatment:

1. **What You Need**: A clean spoolie brush or cotton swab and a small amount of castor oil.
2. **Instructions**: Dip the applicator into the oil, removing any excess to avoid over-application. Gently brush onto your lashes and brows before bedtime.
3. **Safety Tip**: Avoid contact with the eyes. Use a minimal amount to prevent any irritation and keep the treatment focused on hair growth.

Thickening Eyebrow and Eyelash Growth Serum

Purpose/Benefits: Encourages growth for thicker, fuller eyebrows and lashes.

Ingredients:

- 1 teaspoon castor oil
- 1 teaspoon vitamin E oil

Tools/Equipment:

- Small container with brush applicator

Instructions:

1. Combine castor oil and vitamin E oil.
2. Apply sparingly to lashes and brows with the brush.

Application Tips:

- Apply nightly for best results.

Storage and Shelf Life:

- Store in a cool, dry place. Shelf life is 6 months.

Safety Notes:

- Avoid direct contact with eyes.

DIY Hair Masks and Treatments: For Growth, Strength, and Scalp Health

Here are a few easy-to-make DIY hair masks and treatments to support growth, strength, and scalp health, all using the power of castor oil.

Shine-Enhancing Rinse for Dull Hair

Purpose/Benefits: Adds shine and luster to dull hair with castor oil and apple cider vinegar.

Ingredients:

- 1 teaspoon castor oil
- 1 tablespoon apple cider vinegar
- 1 cup warm water

Tools/Equipment:

- Spray bottle or bowl

Instructions:

1. Mix all ingredients in a bowl.
2. Apply to hair after shampooing, focusing on the lengths.

Application Tips:

- Rinse out with cool water after 5 minutes. Use once a week.

Storage and Shelf Life:

- Prepare fresh for each use.

Safety Notes:

- Avoid the eyes as vinegar may cause stinging.

Moisturizing Scalp Treatment for Dry, Flaky Skin

Purpose/Benefits: Hydrates and soothes a dry, flaky scalp.

Ingredients:

- 1 tablespoon castor oil
- 1 tablespoon avocado oil
- 5 drops lavender essential oil (optional)

Tools/Equipment:

- Small bowl

Instructions:

1. Combine all ingredients in the bowl.
2. Apply to the scalp, massaging gently.

Application Tips:

- Leave on for 20 minutes before rinsing. Use weekly for best results.

Storage and Shelf Life:

- Store in a cool, dark place. Use within 3 months.

Safety Notes:

- Do a patch test for any sensitivities.

Heat Protectant Serum for Styling

Purpose/Benefits: Protects hair from heat damage during styling.

Ingredients:

- 1 teaspoon castor oil
- 1 teaspoon grapeseed oil

Tools/Equipment:

- Small container with dropper

Instructions:

1. Mix castor oil and grapeseed oil in a container.
2. Apply a few drops to damp hair before styling.

Application Tips:

- Use only a small amount to avoid a greasy look.

Storage and Shelf Life:

- Store in a cool place for up to 6 months.

Safety Notes:

- Avoid applying directly to the scalp if prone to oiliness.

Scalp Detox Oil Treatment

Purpose/Benefits: Removes buildup and refreshes the scalp.

Ingredients:

- 1 tablespoon castor oil
- 1 tablespoon jojoba oil
- 5 drops lemon essential oil

Tools/Equipment:

- Small bowl

Instructions:

1. Mix oils in a bowl.
2. Massage into the scalp, leaving on for 15 minutes before washing.

Application Tips:

- Use once a month to detox the scalp.

Storage and Shelf Life:

- Store for up to 3 months in a dark place.

Safety Notes:

- Avoid lemon oil exposure to sunlight as it can increase sensitivity.

Natural Highlight Enhancer for Brighter Hair

Purpose/Benefits: Brings out natural highlights, especially in lighter hair tones.

Ingredients:

- 1 tablespoon castor oil
- 1 tablespoon chamomile tea (strongly brewed and cooled)

Tools/Equipment:

- Small spray bottle

Instructions:

1. Mix castor oil and chamomile tea in the spray bottle.
2. Spray onto hair, focusing on areas with natural highlights.

Application Tips:

- Leave on for 30 minutes in sunlight, then rinse. Use as needed.

Storage and Shelf Life:

- Store in the refrigerator for up to 1 week.

Safety Notes:

- Limit sunlight exposure if prone to sun sensitivity.

Castor Oil Pre-Wash Hair Treatment

Purpose/Benefits: Prepares hair for washing, enhancing manageability and softness.

Ingredients:

- 1 tablespoon castor oil
- 1 tablespoon coconut oil

Tools/Equipment:

- Small bowl

Instructions:

1. Mix castor oil and coconut oil in a bowl.
2. Apply to dry hair, focusing on the ends and any dry areas.

Application Tips:

- Leave on for 15-20 minutes before shampooing. Use once a week.

Storage and Shelf Life:

- Prepare fresh for each use.

Safety Notes:

- Avoid applying to the scalp if prone to oiliness.

Overnight Castor Oil Hair Wrap for Intensive Hydration

Purpose/Benefits: Provides deep hydration and softness to hair overnight.

Ingredients:

- 2 tablespoons castor oil
- 1 tablespoon olive oil

Tools/Equipment:

- Shower cap or towel
- Small bowl

Instructions:

1. Mix castor oil and olive oil in a bowl.
2. Apply evenly through hair, focusing on dry areas.

Application Tips:

- Cover with a shower cap or towel, and leave on overnight. Rinse in the morning.

Storage and Shelf Life:

- Prepare fresh each time.

Safety Notes:

- Protect bedding with a towel or shower cap.

Curl Defining Cream for Wavy and Curly Hair

Purpose/Benefits: Enhances and defines curls with castor oil's moisturizing properties.

Ingredients:

- 1 tablespoon castor oil
- 1 tablespoon shea butter (softened)
- 1 tablespoon aloe vera gel

Tools/Equipment:

- Small bowl

Instructions:

1. Combine castor oil, shea butter, and aloe vera gel in a bowl.
2. Mix until smooth and apply to damp hair.

Application Tips:

- Scrunch into curls and allow to air dry. Use as needed.

Storage and Shelf Life:

- Store in a cool place for up to 1 month.

Safety Notes:

- Avoid roots if prone to oiliness.

Each recipe provides an easy way to incorporate castor oil into your hair care routine, offering targeted benefits for growth, moisture, and scalp health.

Health and Wellness Applications

Pain and Inflammation Relief: Joint and Muscle Pain, Arthritis Relief

Castor oil is a go-to remedy for easing joint and muscle pain, especially for those with arthritis or chronic discomfort. Thanks to its natural anti-inflammatory properties, castor oil can help soothe sore areas, reduce inflammation, and provide a sense of relaxation when applied topically.

Application Tips:

- **Direct Application**: Gently massage a small amount of warm castor oil into the affected area, using circular motions to promote relaxation. Leave the oil on for at least 20-30 minutes, allowing it to absorb into the skin and work its magic.
- **Enhanced Warm Compress**: To boost effectiveness, apply a warm compress over the oiled area. Simply place a warm, damp cloth on the area, letting the heat drive the oil deeper into the skin. Repeat this treatment as needed to help alleviate discomfort and stiffness.

Anti-Inflammatory Joint Soak for Arthritis Relief

Purpose/Benefits: Soothes arthritis pain and reduces inflammation through a warm bath soak.

Ingredients:

- 1 tablespoon castor oil
- 1 cup Epsom salts
- 5 drops frankincense essential oil

Tools/Equipment:

- Bathtub

Instructions:

1. Mix all ingredients in a warm bath.
2. Soak for 15-20 minutes, focusing on affected joints.

Application Tips:

- Use 2-3 times per week for best results.

Storage and Shelf Life:

- Prepare fresh for each use.

Safety Notes:

- Not recommended if pregnant without consulting a healthcare provider.

Castor Oil Joint Pain Relief Balm

Purpose/Benefits: Eases joint and muscle pain with a soothing blend of castor oil and menthol.

Ingredients:

- 2 tablespoons castor oil
- 1 tablespoon coconut oil
- 5-6 drops menthol oil
- 1 tablespoon beeswax

Tools/Equipment:

- Small glass jar
- Double boiler or microwave-safe bowl

Instructions:

1. In a double boiler, melt the beeswax and coconut oil together.
2. Stir in the castor oil and menthol oil until well combined.
3. Pour into a glass jar and allow to cool.

Application Tips:

- Apply a small amount to sore joints as needed. Massage gently for best results.

Storage and Shelf Life:

- Store in a cool, dark place for up to 3 months.

Safety Notes:

- Perform a patch test before use, especially for sensitive skin.

Anti-Inflammatory Castor Oil Compress for Sore Muscles

Purpose/Benefits: Reduces muscle soreness and inflammation post-activity.

Ingredients:

- 2 tablespoons castor oil
- 1 soft cloth or cotton pad
- Hot water bottle or heating pad

Tools/Equipment:

- Small bowl

Instructions:

1. Soak the cloth in castor oil and wring out excess.
2. Place the cloth over sore muscles and cover with a hot water bottle.

Application Tips:

- Apply for 20-30 minutes after exercise or strenuous activity.

Storage and Shelf Life:

- Prepare fresh for each use.

Safety Notes:

- Avoid direct contact with open wounds.

Circulation-Boosting Leg Massage Oil

Purpose/Benefits: Improves circulation in the legs, ideal for relieving discomfort in those with limited movement.

Ingredients:

- 1 tablespoon castor oil
- 2 drops rosemary essential oil
- 2 drops juniper essential oil

Tools/Equipment:

- Small container

Instructions:

1. Mix oils in the container.
2. Massage onto legs in upward motions.

Application Tips:

- Use daily for best results, especially after prolonged periods of sitting or standing.

Storage and Shelf Life:

- Store in a cool place for up to 3 months.

Safety Notes:

- Perform a patch test for sensitive skin.

Hand and Foot Soother for Sore Joints and Stiffness

Purpose/Benefits: Relieves joint stiffness and provides soothing comfort for hands and feet.

Ingredients:

- 2 tablespoons castor oil
- 1 tablespoon shea butter
- 5 drops eucalyptus essential oil

Tools/Equipment:

- Small glass jar
- Double boiler

Instructions:

1. Melt shea butter in a double boiler, then stir in castor oil and eucalyptus oil.
2. Pour into a glass jar and allow to cool.

Application Tips:

- Massage onto hands and feet, focusing on sore areas.

Storage and Shelf Life:

- Store in a cool, dark place for up to 3 months.

Safety Notes:

- For external use only. Patch test before applying.

Anti-Stress Relaxation Massage Oil Blend

Purpose/Benefits: Promotes relaxation and helps alleviate stress with a calming massage oil.

Ingredients:

- 1 tablespoon castor oil
- 3 drops lavender essential oil
- 2 drops chamomile essential oil

Tools/Equipment:

- Small container

Instructions:

1. Combine all oils in the container.
2. Massage onto shoulders, neck, or any tense areas.

Application Tips:

- Use after a long day to unwind, as part of a bedtime routine.

Storage and Shelf Life:

- Store in a cool, dark place for up to 3 months.

Safety Notes:

Perform a patch test if you have sensitive skin.

Digestive Health and Constipation Relief: Natural Laxative Effects

Known for its natural laxative properties, castor oil is often used to relieve occasional constipation by gently stimulating the digestive system. When used correctly, it can provide relief from discomfort and promote digestive health.

Safe Usage Guidelines:

- **Dosage:** For adults, a typical dose is about 1-2 teaspoons of castor oil taken on an empty stomach. Effects usually occur within 2-6 hours, so it's best to plan accordingly.
- **Caution:** Castor oil should only be used internally under guidance, especially for those with sensitive stomachs or digestive conditions. If unsure, always consult a healthcare provider before internal use to ensure safe and appropriate application.

Digestive Health Tonic for Occasional Constipation

Purpose/Benefits: Supports digestion and relieves occasional constipation.

Ingredients:

- 1 teaspoon castor oil (food-grade)

Instructions:

1. Take 1 teaspoon of castor oil in the morning, preferably on an empty stomach.

Application Tips:

- Use as needed, no more than once a day.

Storage and Shelf Life:

- Store the castor oil in a cool, dark place.

Safety Notes:

- Consult with a healthcare provider before using internally, especially for children and pregnant individuals.

Castor Oil Pack for Liver Detox and Lymphatic Support

Purpose/Benefits: Supports liver detoxification and lymphatic drainage.

Ingredients:

- 2 tablespoons castor oil
- Cotton flannel or soft cloth
- Heating pad or hot water bottle

Tools/Equipment:

- Plastic wrap (optional)

Instructions:

1. Soak the cloth in castor oil and apply it to the abdomen.
2. Cover with plastic wrap if desired, and place a heating pad on top.

Application Tips:

- Use for 30-60 minutes, once or twice a week.

Storage and Shelf Life:

- Prepare fresh each time.

Safety Notes:

- Avoid use if pregnant without consulting a healthcare provider.

Detoxification and Lymphatic Drainage: Castor Oil Packs for Detox

Castor oil packs are a gentle yet powerful way to stimulate detoxification and support lymphatic drainage, helping the body eliminate toxins and promote overall well-being. These packs encourage improved circulation, liver support, and a natural detox process.

How to Use Castor Oil Packs:

1. **Materials Needed**: Castor oil, a piece of flannel or cloth, plastic wrap, and a heating pad or hot water bottle.

2. **Preparation**: Soak the cloth in castor oil, ensuring it is saturated but not dripping. Place it on your abdomen or liver area.
3. **Application**: Cover the cloth with plastic wrap to prevent leaks, then place a heating pad on top for warmth. Leave the pack on for 30-45 minutes, relaxing while the castor oil promotes circulation and detox.
4. **Aftercare**: Remove the pack, store it in a sealed bag (it can be reused a few times), and gently clean the skin with warm water.

Regular use of castor oil packs may offer gentle detox benefits, helping you feel revitalized and refreshed.

Immune Support: Enhancing Lymph Flow and Fighting Infections

Castor oil can be a supportive addition to your immune health routine, as it promotes lymph flow and circulation, essential for a resilient immune system. Its antimicrobial properties also help protect against common pathogens, supporting overall health.

Usage Tips for Immune Health:

- **Lymph Node Application**: Apply a small amount of castor oil to areas with major lymph nodes, like the neck or armpits, and gently massage. This may help improve lymphatic drainage and circulation.
- **Regular Immune Support Massage**: Incorporate castor oil into a gentle self-massage routine. Regular massages with castor oil can stimulate the immune system naturally and provide an added layer of wellness support.

<u>Immune-Boosting Chest Rub</u>

Purpose/Benefits: Supports respiratory health and immunity with a eucalyptus chest rub.

Ingredients:

- 1 tablespoon castor oil
- 5 drops eucalyptus essential oil
- 3 drops tea tree oil

Tools/Equipment:

- Small glass jar

Instructions:

1. Combine all oils in the jar.
2. Rub a small amount onto the chest as needed.

Application Tips:

- Use before bed to support respiratory health during cold and flu season.

Storage and Shelf Life:

- Store for up to 3 months in a cool place.

Safety Notes:

- Not suitable for children under 6 years.

DIY Health Remedies: Recipes for Headache Relief, Sinus Congestion, and General Wellness

Here are some easy DIY recipes using castor oil to address everyday health concerns like headaches, sinus congestion, and overall wellness.

Castor Oil Cold and Flu Chest Compress

Purpose/Benefits: Provides comfort and relief for chest congestion during cold and flu season.

Ingredients:

- 2 tablespoons castor oil
- 5 drops eucalyptus essential oil
- Soft cloth or flannel
- Hot water bottle or heating pad

Tools/Equipment:

- Small bowl

Instructions:

1. Mix castor oil and eucalyptus oil in a bowl.
2. Soak the cloth in the mixture and wring out the excess.
3. Place the cloth over the chest, then apply a hot water bottle or heating pad on top.

Application Tips:

- Leave compress on for 15-20 minutes, once or twice daily as needed.

Storage and Shelf Life:

- Prepare fresh each time.

Safety Notes:

- Not suitable for children under 6. Avoid direct contact with eyes.

Castor Oil Remedy for Menstrual Cramps

Purpose/Benefits: Eases menstrual cramps and abdominal discomfort with a soothing massage oil.

Ingredients:

- 2 tablespoons castor oil
- 3 drops lavender essential oil
- 2 drops clary sage essential oil

Tools/Equipment:

- Small glass container

Instructions:

1. Mix castor oil with lavender and clary sage essential oils in a container.

2. Massage onto the lower abdomen.

Application Tips:

- Use during cramping, applying a warm compress over the area after massage if desired.

Storage and Shelf Life:

- Store in a cool place for up to 3 months.

Safety Notes:

- Consult a healthcare provider if pregnant or breastfeeding.

Digestive Massage Oil for Bloating Relief

Purpose/Benefits: Helps reduce bloating and supports digestion through a gentle abdominal massage.

Ingredients:

- 1 tablespoon castor oil
- 3 drops ginger essential oil
- 3 drops peppermint essential oil

Tools/Equipment:

- Small container

Instructions:

1. Mix all oils in the container.
2. Massage onto the abdomen in a clockwise motion.

Application Tips:

- Use daily or as needed for digestive support.

Storage and Shelf Life:

- Store for up to 3 months in a cool, dark place.

Safety Notes:

- For external use only.

Sinus Relief Steam Treatment with Castor Oil

Purpose/Benefits: Clears sinuses and eases congestion through steam inhalation.

Ingredients:

- 1 teaspoon castor oil
- 2 drops eucalyptus essential oil
- Hot water

Tools/Equipment:

- Bowl
- Towel

Instructions:

1. Add castor oil and essential oil to a bowl of hot water.
2. Drape a towel over your head and inhale the steam for 5-10 minutes.

Application Tips:

- Use once daily as needed.

Storage and Shelf Life:

- Prepare fresh each time.

Safety Notes:

- Avoid direct eye contact with steam.

Migraine and Headache Relief Massage Oil

Purpose/Benefits: Provides natural headache relief when massaged onto temples and neck.

Ingredients:

- 1 tablespoon castor oil
- 2-3 drops peppermint essential oil
- 2-3 drops lavender essential oil

Tools/Equipment:

- Small container

Instructions:

1. Mix castor oil with essential oils in a container.
2. Massage onto temples and neck.

Application Tips:

- Apply gently whenever experiencing headache symptoms.

Storage and Shelf Life:

- Store in a cool, dark place for up to 6 months.

Safety Notes:

- Avoid contact with eyes.

Castor Oil Temple Rub for Tension Headaches

Purpose/Benefits: Relieves headache tension with a soothing temple massage.

Ingredients:

- 1 teaspoon castor oil
- 2 drops peppermint essential oil

Tools/Equipment:

- Small container

Instructions:

1. Mix castor oil and peppermint oil.

Application Tips:

- Apply a small amount to temples and gently massage.

Storage and Shelf Life:

- Use within 3 months.

Safety Notes:

- Avoid contact with eyes.

Castor Oil Earache Relief Remedy

Purpose/Benefits: Provides gentle, natural relief for mild earaches.

Ingredients:

- 1 teaspoon castor oil (slightly warmed)

Tools/Equipment:

- Cotton ball

Instructions:

1. Slightly warm the castor oil (test for temperature).
2. Dab a small amount onto a cotton ball and place it gently in the outer ear.

Application Tips:

- Use once daily as needed for relief.

Storage and Shelf Life:

- Prepare fresh each time.

Safety Notes:

- Do not apply directly into the ear canal. Consult a healthcare provider for severe ear pain.

Wound and Minor Cuts Healing Ointment

Purpose/Benefits: Supports the healing of minor cuts and scrapes.

Ingredients:

- 1 tablespoon castor oil
- 1 tablespoon coconut oil
- 5 drops tea tree essential oil

Tools/Equipment:

- Small jar

Instructions:

1. Mix all ingredients in the jar.
2. Apply a small amount to minor cuts.

Application Tips:

- Use as needed to protect and heal minor wounds.

Storage and Shelf Life:

- Store for up to 3 months in a cool place.

Safety Notes:

- Avoid use on deep wounds or infections.

Sleep-Inducing Castor Oil Foot Rub

Purpose/Benefits: Promotes restful sleep with a soothing castor oil and lavender blend.

Ingredients:

- 1 tablespoon castor oil
- 2 drops lavender essential oil

Tools/Equipment:

- Small container

Instructions:

1. Mix castor oil with lavender oil.
2. Massage onto the bottoms of your feet before bed.

Application Tips:

- Apply nightly for best results.

Storage and Shelf Life:

- Store in a cool, dark place for up to 3 months.

Safety Notes:

- For external use only.

Anti-Itch Remedy for Bug Bites and Skin Irritations

Purpose/Benefits: Relieves itchiness from bug bites and skin irritations.

Ingredients:

- 1 tablespoon castor oil
- 3 drops chamomile essential oil

Tools/Equipment:

- Small container

Instructions:

1. Combine oils in the container.
2. Dab onto bug bites or itchy areas.

Application Tips:

- Reapply as needed for itch relief.

Storage and Shelf Life:

- Store in a cool, dark place for up to 3 months.

Safety Notes:

- Avoid broken skin.

Stress Relief and Relaxation

Massage Oil for Stress Relief: Relaxing Muscles and Easing Tension

Castor oil's smooth texture and rich moisturizing properties make it an ideal choice for massage, especially when you're looking to ease stress and release muscle tension after a long day. Known for its thickness and natural warmth, castor oil glides smoothly on the skin, providing a calming effect while allowing deeper muscle relaxation. The act of massaging with castor oil can improve circulation, reduce physical tension, and promote a sense of tranquility.

How to Use Castor Oil for Massage:

- **Warming the Oil**: Warm a small amount of castor oil in your hands or gently heat it until it's comfortably warm. The warmth enhances relaxation and helps the oil penetrate the muscles more effectively.
- **Application**: Apply the warm castor oil to areas with tight muscles—such as the neck, shoulders, or back—using gentle, circular motions to relieve tension. Take slow, deep breaths during the massage to help your body and mind unwind.
- **Adding Essential Oils**: For added relaxation, mix a few drops of lavender or chamomile essential oil into the castor oil. These scents are known for their calming properties and can enhance the overall stress-relief effect.

A regular castor oil massage can become a comforting ritual, encouraging relaxation and providing relief from daily stresses.

Castor Oil Calming Massage Oil for Full-Body Relaxation

Purpose/Benefits: A relaxing full-body massage oil that promotes calm and relaxation through gentle aromatherapy.

Ingredients:

- 2 tablespoons castor oil
- 5 drops lavender essential oil
- 3 drops chamomile essential oil

Tools/Equipment:

- Small mixing bowl
- Massage bottle (optional)

Instructions:

1. Combine castor oil, lavender oil, and chamomile oil in the mixing bowl.
2. Transfer the mixture to a massage bottle if desired.

Application Tips:

- Apply with gentle strokes for a full-body massage or target specific areas to relieve tension.

Storage and Shelf Life:

- Store in a cool, dark place for up to 3 months.

Safety Notes:

- Perform a patch test if you have sensitive skin.

Foot Massage Oil for Stress Relief

Purpose/Benefits: A calming foot massage oil that relaxes tired feet and relieves stress.

Ingredients:

- 1 tablespoon castor oil
- 3 drops peppermint essential oil
- 2 drops rosemary essential oil

Tools/Equipment:

- Small container

Instructions:

1. Mix oils in the container.

Application Tips:

- Massage into feet, focusing on the arches and heels.

Storage and Shelf Life:

- Lasts up to 3 months in a cool place.

Safety Notes:

Avoid contact with eyes and broken skin.

Hand and Wrist Relaxation Oil for Tension Relief

Purpose/Benefits: Relieves hand and wrist tension, perfect for frequent computer users.

Ingredients:

- 1 teaspoon castor oil
- 2 drops lemon balm essential oil
- 2 drops eucalyptus essential oil

Tools/Equipment:

- Small container

Instructions:

1. Mix all oils in the container.

Application Tips:

- Massage into hands and wrists as needed.

Storage and Shelf Life:

- Lasts up to 3 months.

Safety Notes:

- Patch test for sensitive skin.

Aromatherapy and Calming Blends: Castor Oil with Essential Oils for Anxiety Relief

Combining castor oil with calming essential oils opens up a range of soothing aromatherapy options, perfect for reducing anxiety and creating a peaceful atmosphere. Castor oil acts as a gentle carrier oil, delivering the benefits of essential oils while nourishing the skin.

Creating a Calming Blend:

- **Essential Oils to Use**: Lavender, chamomile, and eucalyptus are particularly effective for relaxation and can be easily blended with castor oil for anxiety relief.
- **Basic Blend Recipe**: Mix 1 tablespoon of castor oil with 3-4 drops of your preferred essential oil(s). This mixture can be used as a topical application, or you can apply it to pulse points (like wrists or temples) for a calming effect.
- **Inhalation or Diffusion**: Alternatively, place a few drops of the blend on a cloth and inhale deeply, or use it with a diffuser to create a tranquil environment in your home.

Castor Oil Calming Diffuser Blend

Purpose/Benefits: Creates a peaceful, calming atmosphere.

Ingredients:

- 5 drops sandalwood essential oil
- 3 drops vanilla essential oil

Tools/Equipment:

- Essential oil diffuser

Instructions:

1. Add oils to diffuser with water as directed.

Application Tips:

- Use during meditation or relaxation time.

Safety Notes:

- Follow diffuser safety guidelines.

Anxiety-Reducing Castor Oil Inhalation Blend

Purpose/Benefits: Provides quick, calming relief during stressful moments.

Ingredients:

- 1 teaspoon castor oil
- 5 drops lavender essential oil

Tools/Equipment:

- Inhaler or tissue

Instructions:

1. Add lavender oil to castor oil.
2. Inhale directly from the tissue or an inhaler.

Application Tips:

- Use during times of heightened anxiety.

Safety Notes:

- Avoid direct skin contact with undiluted essential oils.

Stress-Reducing Eye Pillow with Castor Oil Infusion

Purpose/Benefits: A DIY eye pillow infused with a calming blend for relaxation.

Ingredients:

- 1 tablespoon castor oil
- 3 drops lavender essential oil
- Small muslin or cloth eye pillow

Tools/Equipment:

- Small bowl

Instructions:

1. Mix castor oil and lavender oil in a bowl.
2. Apply a few drops to the exterior of the eye pillow, allowing it to absorb.

Application Tips:

- Place the eye pillow over your eyes during relaxation or meditation.

Storage and Shelf Life:

- Keep the pillow in a cool, dry place; refresh oil mixture as needed.

Safety Notes:

- Ensure oils do not directly touch the eyes.

Anti-Anxiety Castor Oil Pulse Point Roll-On

Purpose/Benefits: A calming roll-on blend to apply to pulse points during moments of stress.

Ingredients:

- 1 teaspoon castor oil
- 5 drops lavender essential oil
- 3 drops bergamot essential oil

Tools/Equipment:

- Small roll-on bottle

Instructions:

1. Combine castor oil with essential oils in the roll-on bottle.
2. Secure the cap and shake gently to mix.

Application Tips:

- Apply to pulse points on wrists, temples, or neck as needed.

Storage and Shelf Life:

- Lasts up to 6 months.

Safety Notes:

- Avoid contact with sensitive areas, such as eyes.

Aromatherapy with castor oil and essential oils provides a gentle, comforting experience that can ease tension and promote emotional balance.

DIY Relaxation Recipes: Stress Relief Oils, Bath Blends, and Sleep Aids

Enhance your relaxation routine with these simple, DIY recipes using castor oil to help you unwind, relieve stress, and promote restful sleep.

Castor Oil Stress-Relief Body Spray

Purpose/Benefits: A light body spray with a calming scent to reduce stress.

Ingredients:

- 1 teaspoon castor oil
- 1 cup distilled water
- 5 drops lavender essential oil
- 3 drops sandalwood essential oil

Tools/Equipment:

- Small spray bottle

Instructions:

1. Combine all ingredients in the spray bottle and shake well.

Application Tips:

- Spritz lightly over the body as needed for stress relief.

Storage and Shelf Life:

- Use within 1 month.

Safety Notes:

- Avoid contact with eyes and face.

Stress-Relief Bath Soak with Castor Oil and Epsom Salt

Purpose/Benefits: A luxurious soak to ease muscle tension and promote relaxation.

Ingredients:

- 1 tablespoon castor oil
- 1 cup Epsom salts
- 5 drops lavender essential oil
- 3 drops eucalyptus essential oil

Tools/Equipment:

- Bathtub

Instructions:

1. Mix castor oil with essential oils.
2. Add the mixture and Epsom salts to a warm bath.

Application Tips:

- Soak for 15-20 minutes for the best results.

Storage and Shelf Life:

- Prepare fresh for each use.

Safety Notes:

- Be cautious of slippery surfaces due to castor oil in the tub.

Calming Face Massage Oil for Stress Relief

Purpose/Benefits: Reduces facial tension and promotes relaxation.

Ingredients:

- 1 teaspoon castor oil
- 2 drops rose essential oil
- 2 drops chamomile essential oil

Tools/Equipment:

- Small container

Instructions:

1. Combine oils in the container.

Application Tips:

- Massage gently over the face and jawline.

Storage and Shelf Life:

- Store for up to 3 months.

Safety Notes:

- Perform a patch test for sensitive skin.

Castor Oil Sleep Balm for Restful Nights

Purpose/Benefits: A soothing balm to calm the senses and prepare for sleep.

Ingredients:

- 1 tablespoon castor oil
- 1 tablespoon coconut oil
- 5 drops valerian essential oil
- 3 drops lavender essential oil

Tools/Equipment:

- Small glass jar

Instructions:

1. Combine all ingredients in the jar and mix well.
2. Store in a cool place.

Application Tips:

- Apply to pulse points before bed.

Storage and Shelf Life:

- Lasts up to 6 months in a cool place.

Safety Notes:

- Avoid if sensitive to valerian.

Tranquil Aromatherapy Pillow Spray with Castor Oil Base

Purpose/Benefits: A pillow spray to help relax the mind before sleep.

Ingredients:

- 1 teaspoon castor oil
- 1 cup distilled water
- 10 drops lavender essential oil
- 5 drops bergamot essential oil

Tools/Equipment:

- Small spray bottle

Instructions:

1. Add castor oil, water, and essential oils to the spray bottle.
2. Shake well before each use.

Application Tips:

- Lightly spray on your pillow before sleep.

Storage and Shelf Life:

- Use within 1 month.

Safety Notes:

- Avoid direct contact with the face and eyes.

Sleep-Enhancing Castor Oil Bedtime Rub

Purpose/Benefits: A soothing bedtime rub to promote restful sleep.

Ingredients:

- 1 tablespoon castor oil
- 3 drops vetiver essential oil
- 2 drops chamomile essential oil

Tools/Equipment:

- Small mixing bowl
- Glass jar for storage

Instructions:

1. Mix castor oil, vetiver oil, and chamomile oil in the bowl until well combined.
2. Transfer the mixture to a glass jar.

Application Tips:

- Rub a small amount on your chest and neck before bed.

Storage and Shelf Life:

- Store in a cool, dark place for up to 6 months.

Safety Notes:

Avoid contact with eyes and broken skin.

Castor Oil Bath Melts with Lavender and Chamomile

Purpose/Benefits: DIY bath melts for a relaxing, hydrating bath experience.

Ingredients:

- 1 tablespoon castor oil
- 1 tablespoon shea butter
- 5 drops lavender essential oil
- 3 drops chamomile essential oil

Tools/Equipment:

- Small silicone mold (for shaping melts)

Instructions:

1. Melt castor oil and shea butter together in a microwave or double boiler.
2. Stir in lavender and chamomile oils, then pour the mixture into the mold.
3. Let it cool and solidify.

Application Tips:

- Drop one melt into a warm bath, allowing it to dissolve.

Storage and Shelf Life:

- Store in a cool, dark place for up to 3 months.

Safety Notes:

- Be cautious of slippery surfaces in the bath.

Castor Oil Bath Bombs for Stress Relief

Purpose/Benefits: DIY bath bombs with calming scents for a relaxing bath experience.

Ingredients:

- 1 tablespoon castor oil
- 1 cup baking soda
- 1/2 cup citric acid
- 5 drops lavender essential oil
- 3 drops chamomile essential oil

Tools/Equipment:

- Mixing bowl
- Bath bomb molds

Instructions:

1. Mix baking soda and citric acid.
2. Add castor oil and essential oils, mixing well.
3. Press the mixture into molds and let set.

Application Tips:

- Drop one bomb into a warm bath and enjoy.

Storage and Shelf Life:

- Store in a dry place for up to 3 months.

Safety Notes:

- Handle carefully, as bath bombs may be fragile.

These DIY recipes offer a variety of ways to incorporate castor oil into your self-care routine, allowing you to enjoy relaxation and peace at your convenience. Whether you prefer a soothing bath, a targeted massage, or a calming aroma, castor oil can be a wonderful companion in your journey toward daily stress relief and restful nights.

Baby and Children's Care

Diaper Rash Treatment: Safe and Gentle Soothing for Sensitive Skin

Castor oil's natural moisturizing and anti-inflammatory properties make it an ideal choice for soothing diaper rash in babies. Its gentle touch helps reduce redness, irritation, and discomfort, offering a chemical-free alternative to commercial diaper creams. Castor oil's mild nature ensures that it's safe for even the most sensitive skin, providing relief without harsh additives.

How to Use Castor Oil for Diaper Rash:

- **Preparation**: Begin with clean, dry skin. After changing the diaper and gently patting the area dry, apply a thin layer of castor oil to the affected skin.
- **Application**: Use just a small amount and spread it evenly. The oil creates a protective barrier that keeps moisture away, soothing irritation and helping the skin to heal.
- **Routine**: Consider applying castor oil as part of each diaper change for consistent relief and prevention of further irritation.

Diaper Rash Soothing Balm with Castor Oil

Purpose/Benefits: A gentle balm to calm diaper rash and prevent irritation.

Ingredients:

- 1 tablespoon castor oil (organic, cold-pressed)
- 1 tablespoon coconut oil
- 2 drops chamomile essential oil (optional)

Tools/Equipment:

- Small mixing bowl
- Storage container

Instructions:

1. Combine castor oil and coconut oil in the mixing bowl.
2. Add chamomile oil if using, and mix well.
3. Transfer to a storage container.

Application Tips:

- Apply a thin layer to clean, dry skin at each diaper change.

Storage and Shelf Life:

- Store in a cool, dry place for up to 3 months.

Safety Notes:

- Avoid contact with eyes. Test a small area for sensitivity.

<u>**Castor Oil Diaper Barrier Cream**</u>

Purpose/Benefits: A barrier cream to protect skin from diaper rash.

Ingredients:

- 1 tablespoon castor oil
- 1 teaspoon zinc oxide
- 1 teaspoon coconut oil

Tools/Equipment:

- Mixing bowl
- Small container

Instructions:

1. Mix all ingredients in the bowl until smooth.
2. Transfer to a container for storage.

Application Tips:

- Apply a thin layer during diaper changes to protect skin.

Storage and Shelf Life:

- Store in a cool place; lasts up to 3 months.

Safety Notes:

- Test on a small area first to ensure no reaction.

Castor oil's soothing qualities make it an excellent natural solution for easing diaper rash and keeping your baby comfortable.

Minor Skin Irritations: Healing Small Scrapes, Cuts, and Insect Bites

Castor oil can also be a gentle, effective remedy for minor skin irritations in children, including small scrapes, cuts, or insect bites. Its antibacterial and anti-inflammatory properties help protect the skin, reduce swelling, and promote healing, offering relief without the sting of more astringent products.

How to Use Castor Oil for Minor Skin Irritations:

- **Preparation**: Before applying castor oil, clean the affected area gently with mild soap and water, then pat dry.
- **Application**: Dab a small amount of castor oil onto the irritated area with a cotton swab or clean fingertip. Avoid applying too much to keep the area breathable.
- **Reapplication**: Reapply as needed, particularly after washing or bathing, to maintain moisture and support healing.

Healing Ointment for Minor Cuts and Scrapes

Purpose/Benefits: A soothing ointment to help minor scrapes heal quickly.

Ingredients:

- 1 tablespoon castor oil
- 1 teaspoon calendula oil

Tools/Equipment:

- Small mixing bowl
- Storage container

Instructions:

1. Mix castor oil and calendula oil in a bowl.
2. Transfer to a container for storage.

Application Tips:

- Apply a small amount to clean cuts or scrapes as needed.

Storage and Shelf Life:

- Keep in a cool place for up to 6 months.

Safety Notes:

- Perform a patch test for sensitivity.

Castor Oil and Aloe Soothing Gel for Bug Bites

Purpose/Benefits: A soothing gel to relieve itching and irritation from bug bites.

Ingredients:

- 1 tablespoon castor oil
- 1 tablespoon aloe vera gel

Tools/Equipment:

- Small mixing bowl
- Container with lid

Instructions:

1. Mix castor oil with aloe vera gel.
2. Store in a container with a lid.

Application Tips:

- Dab onto bug bites to relieve itching.

Storage and Shelf Life:

- Keep refrigerated; lasts up to 1 month.

Safety Notes:

- Safe for use on children; avoid eyes.

Natural Castor Oil Sunscreen Balm for Sensitive Skin

Purpose/Benefits: A gentle sunscreen balm for sensitive baby skin, protecting from the sun.

Ingredients:

- 1 tablespoon castor oil
- 1 teaspoon zinc oxide (non-nano)
- 1 teaspoon coconut oil

Tools/Equipment:

- Mixing bowl
- Small container

Instructions:

1. Mix all ingredients thoroughly in the bowl.
2. Transfer to a container for storage.

Application Tips:

- Apply a thin layer to exposed skin before sun exposure.

Storage and Shelf Life:

- Store in a cool place; lasts up to 3 months.

Safety Notes:

- Suitable for babies over 6 months. Reapply as needed.

Castor Oil Cradle Cap Scalp Treatment

Purpose/Benefits: A gentle treatment to soften and remove cradle cap.

Ingredients:

- 1 tablespoon castor oil
- 1 tablespoon coconut oil

Tools/Equipment:

- Small bowl
- Soft baby brush or washcloth

Instructions:

1. Mix castor oil and coconut oil in the bowl.
2. Gently massage onto the scalp and leave for 10 minutes.
3. Use a soft baby brush or washcloth to remove softened flakes.

Application Tips:

- Use 2-3 times a week until cradle cap clears.

Storage and Shelf Life:

- Store in a cool place for up to 3 months.

Safety Notes:

- Avoid contact with eyes.

By using castor oil on small skin irritations, you can provide comfort and gentle healing for your child's scrapes and bites in a natural way.

Family-Friendly Applications: General Wellness and Skin Care for Children

Beyond targeted remedies, castor oil can be incorporated into daily routines to keep children's skin soft, hydrated, and comfortable. Its gentle, moisturizing properties make it suitable for a variety of uses, from keeping skin nourished to supporting bedtime relaxation.

Ideas for Using Castor Oil in Family Wellness:

- **Bedtime Massage**: For a calming bedtime ritual, warm a small amount of castor oil in your hands and gently massage it onto your child's back, arms, or legs. This helps relax muscles and provides a sense of comfort before sleep.
- **Moisturizing Dry Areas**: Apply castor oil to areas prone to dryness, like elbows, knees, and cheeks. It provides long-lasting hydration and protection against chafing or dryness, especially in colder months.
- **Gentle Lip and Skin Care**: Dab a tiny amount on lips or any dry patches, ensuring smooth and soft skin without exposure to chemicals.

Castor Oil Rash Relief Cream for Skin Sensitivities

Purpose/Benefits: A gentle cream to soothe rashes and irritation from sensitive skin conditions.

Ingredients:

- 1 tablespoon castor oil
- 1 tablespoon shea butter
- 1 teaspoon calendula oil

Tools/Equipment:

- Small mixing bowl
- Storage container

Instructions:

1. Blend castor oil, shea butter, and calendula oil until smooth.
2. Store in a container with a lid.

Application Tips:

- Apply a thin layer to affected areas as needed.

Storage and Shelf Life:

- Lasts up to 3 months when stored in a cool place.

Safety Notes:

- Perform a patch test for sensitivity, especially on sensitive skin.

Moisturizing Castor Oil Lip Balm for Chapped Lips

Purpose/Benefits: A hydrating, natural lip balm for chapped lips, perfect for kids.

Ingredients:

- 1 tablespoon castor oil

- 1 teaspoon beeswax
- 1 drop honey (optional)

Tools/Equipment:

- Small saucepan
- Lip balm container

Instructions:

1. Melt beeswax in a small saucepan over low heat.
2. Add castor oil and honey, stirring until smooth.
3. Pour into lip balm container and allow to cool.

Application Tips:

- Apply as needed to hydrate and protect lips.

Storage and Shelf Life:

- Store in a cool, dry place; lasts up to 6 months.

Safety Notes:

- Avoid if allergic to beeswax.

Gentle Castor Oil Cleanser for Sensitive Skin

Purpose/Benefits: A mild cleanser to remove dirt without irritating delicate skin.

Ingredients:

- 1 tablespoon castor oil
- 1 tablespoon jojoba oil

Tools/Equipment:

- Small bottle

Instructions:

1. Mix castor oil and jojoba oil in a small bottle.

Application Tips:

- Massage a few drops onto the face, then rinse with warm water.

Storage and Shelf Life:

- Store in a cool place; lasts up to 6 months.

Safety Notes:

- Test on a small area first to ensure no reaction.

Castor Oil and Lavender Sleep Time Massage Oil

Purpose/Benefits: A calming massage oil to help children relax before sleep.

Ingredients:

- 1 tablespoon castor oil
- 2 drops lavender essential oil

Tools/Equipment:

- Small jar or bottle

Instructions:

1. Mix castor oil and lavender oil.
2. Store in a jar or bottle.

Application Tips:

- Massage onto feet or back before bedtime.

Storage and Shelf Life:

- Use within 6 months.

Safety Notes:

- Test on a small area first to ensure no reaction.

Castor Oil and Lavender Bedtime Roll-On

Purpose/Benefits: A calming roll-on to help children relax before bedtime.

Ingredients:

- 1 tablespoon castor oil
- 2 drops lavender essential oil

Tools/Equipment:

- Roll-on bottle

Instructions:

1. Combine castor oil and lavender oil in the roll-on bottle.

Application Tips:

- Roll onto pulse points, like wrists and behind ears, before bedtime.

Storage and Shelf Life:

- Store in a cool place; lasts up to 6 months.

Safety Notes:

- Suitable for children over 6 months; avoid eyes.

Cracked Skin Balm for Baby's Feet and Elbows

Purpose/Benefits: A hydrating balm to soften dry skin areas.

Ingredients:

- 1 tablespoon castor oil
- 1 tablespoon shea butter
- 1 drop chamomile essential oil (optional)

Tools/Equipment:

- Small mixing bowl
- Storage container

Instructions:

1. Mix castor oil and shea butter until smooth.
2. Add chamomile oil if desired, then store.

Application Tips:

- Apply to dry areas like elbows and heels as needed.

Storage and Shelf Life:

- Store in a cool place for up to 3 months.

Safety Notes:

- Test on a small area first for sensitivity.

Gentle Baby Massage Oil for Daily Moisture

Purpose/Benefits: A nourishing oil to keep baby's skin soft after bath time.

Ingredients:

- 1 tablespoon castor oil
- 1 tablespoon sweet almond oil

Tools/Equipment:

- Small bottle or jar

Instructions:

1. Combine both oils and mix well.
2. Store in a bottle.

Application Tips:

- Massage gently onto baby's skin after bathing.

Storage and Shelf Life:

- Store in a cool place for up to 3 months.

Safety Notes:

- Avoid eyes and perform a patch test first.

Castor Oil Teething Relief Balm

Purpose/Benefits: A soothing balm for comforting teething discomfort.

Ingredients:

- 1 tablespoon castor oil
- 1 drop chamomile extract

Tools/Equipment:

- Small container with lid

Instructions:

1. Mix castor oil with chamomile extract.
2. Store in a container with a lid.

Application Tips:

- Gently rub on the outside of cheeks near gums.

Storage and Shelf Life:

- Store for up to 3 months.

Safety Notes:

- Avoid internal use; apply only on cheeks.

Natural Castor Oil Chest Rub for Cold Relief

Purpose/Benefits: A mild rub to help ease congestion during colds.

Ingredients:

- 1 tablespoon castor oil
- 2 drops eucalyptus essential oil (for children over 2 years)

Tools/Equipment:

- Small jar for storage

Instructions:

1. Combine castor oil with eucalyptus oil and mix well.
2. Store in a jar.

Application Tips:

- Rub a small amount onto the chest, avoiding the face.

Storage and Shelf Life:

- Store for up to 6 months.

Safety Notes:

- Eucalyptus oil is suitable for children over 2; avoid for younger children.

Natural Castor Oil Hair Detangler for Kids

Purpose/Benefits: A detangling spray to smooth tangles and make brushing easier.

Ingredients:

- 1 tablespoon castor oil
- 1 cup distilled water
- 1 teaspoon aloe vera gel
- 2 drops lavender essential oil

Tools/Equipment:

- Spray bottle

Instructions:

1. Combine all ingredients in a spray bottle and shake well.

Application Tips:

- Spritz on damp hair, then brush gently to detangle.

Storage and Shelf Life:

- Use within 1 month.

Safety Notes:

- Avoid eyes; suitable for children 2 years and older.

Castor Oil Calming Bath Drops for Fussy Nights

Purpose/Benefits: Soothing bath drops to help calm fussy or overtired children before bed.

Ingredients:

- 1 tablespoon castor oil
- 2 drops lavender essential oil
- 1 drop chamomile essential oil

Tools/Equipment:

- Small dropper bottle

Instructions:

1. Mix castor oil with essential oils.
2. Transfer the blend to a dropper bottle.

Application Tips:

- Add 3-4 drops to warm bath water and swish to mix.

Storage and Shelf Life:

- Store in a cool place; lasts up to 3 months.

Safety Notes:

- Safe for children over 6 months; avoid contact with eyes.

Castor Oil Inhalation Drops for Stuffy Noses

Purpose/Benefits: Drops to help ease nasal congestion safely for young children.

Ingredients:

- 1 teaspoon castor oil
- 1 drop eucalyptus essential oil (for children over 2)

Tools/Equipment:

- Small dropper bottle

Instructions:

1. Combine the oils in a dropper bottle.

Application Tips:

- Place a few drops in a warm bowl of water for inhalation, or dab a small amount near nostrils.

Storage and Shelf Life:

- Store for up to 6 months in a cool place.

Safety Notes:

- Eucalyptus oil is not recommended for children under 2.

Castor Oil and Chamomile Soothing Balm for Growing Pains

Purpose/Benefits: A massage balm for comforting children experiencing growing pains.

Ingredients:

- 1 tablespoon castor oil
- 1 teaspoon chamomile oil

Tools/Equipment:

- Small jar or container

Instructions:

1. Mix castor oil and chamomile oil in a container.

Application Tips:

- Gently massage onto legs before bedtime.

Storage and Shelf Life:

- Store for up to 3 months in a cool place.

Safety Notes:

- Avoid eyes and sensitive areas.

Castor Oil Ear Relief Drops for Ear Discomfort

Purpose/Benefits: A comforting remedy for occasional ear discomfort.

Ingredients:

- 1 teaspoon castor oil
- 1 drop garlic oil (optional, for added antibacterial benefits)

Tools/Equipment:

- Dropper bottle

Instructions:

1. Combine oils in a dropper bottle.

Application Tips:

- Warm slightly, then place 1-2 drops in the affected ear (consult a pediatrician first).

Storage and Shelf Life:

- Store for up to 3 months in a cool place.

Safety Notes:

- Consult with a healthcare provider before use, especially with young children.

With its mild and versatile nature, castor oil is a nurturing addition to family wellness, allowing parents to care for their children's skin naturally and confidently.

Men's Grooming

Beard Care: Conditioning and Softening for Healthy Beard Growth

Castor oil's rich, nourishing properties make it a go-to choice for beard care. Its moisturizing qualities not only soften the beard but also condition the skin underneath, helping to prevent beard itch and dryness. Regular use can lead to a fuller, healthier-looking beard that's easier to manage.

How to Use Castor Oil for Beard Care:

- **Apply to a Clean, Dry Beard**: After washing and drying your beard, warm a few drops of castor oil in your hands and massage it into the beard, reaching the skin underneath.
- **Add Other Oils for Extra Benefits**: Combine castor oil with lighter oils like jojoba or argan to create a nourishing blend that absorbs quickly, leaving the beard soft without feeling greasy.
- **Use Regularly**: Consistent use can reduce itchiness and improve manageability, making your beard softer and more resilient over time.

Castor Oil Beard Softening and Conditioning Serum

Purpose/Benefits: Softens facial hair, reduces itch, and nourishes the skin beneath for a healthier beard.

Ingredients:

- 1 tablespoon castor oil
- 1 tablespoon argan oil
- 2 drops cedarwood essential oil

Tools/Equipment:

- Small bottle with dropper

Instructions:

1. Mix all ingredients in the bottle.
2. Shake gently to combine.

Application Tips:

- Apply a few drops to the beard and massage through to the roots.
- Use daily for best results.

Storage and Shelf Life:

- Store in a cool, dark place; lasts up to 6 months.

Safety Notes:

- Avoid direct contact with eyes.

Daily Beard Oil for Fuller Growth and Shine

Purpose/Benefits: Lightweight oil to add shine and promote fuller beard growth.

Ingredients:

- 1 tablespoon castor oil
- 1 tablespoon jojoba oil
- 3 drops cedarwood essential oil

Tools/Equipment:

- Small dropper bottle

Instructions:

1. Combine all ingredients in the bottle.
2. Shake to blend.

Application Tips:

- Massage a few drops into the beard daily for shine and moisture.

Storage and Shelf Life:

- Keep in a cool, dark place; lasts up to 6 months.

Safety Notes:

- Perform a patch test before full use.

Overnight Beard Growth Treatment with Castor Oil

Purpose/Benefits: A rich blend to promote thicker and faster beard growth overnight.

Ingredients:

- 1 tablespoon castor oil
- 1 teaspoon vitamin E oil

Tools/Equipment:

- Small bottle

Instructions:

1. Mix castor oil and vitamin E oil in the bottle.

Application Tips:

- Apply to beard before bed and wash out in the morning.

Storage and Shelf Life:

- Store in a cool, dark place; lasts up to 6 months.

Safety Notes:

- Avoid direct contact with eyes.

Beard Thickening Oil Blend with Castor Oil and Eucalyptus

Purpose/Benefits: Helps create a fuller, healthier-looking beard.

Ingredients:

- 1 tablespoon castor oil
- 1 tablespoon coconut oil
- 2 drops eucalyptus essential oil

Tools/Equipment:

- Small bottle

Instructions:

1. Mix the oils in a bottle and shake to blend.

Application Tips:

- Massage a few drops into the beard daily.

Storage and Shelf Life:

- Store in a cool, dark place; lasts up to 6 months.

Safety Notes:

- Avoid direct contact with eyes.

Castor Oil Mustache Wax with Hold and Conditioning

Purpose/Benefits: Provides hold for styling while conditioning the mustache.

Ingredients:

- 1 tablespoon castor oil
- 1 tablespoon beeswax
- 1 teaspoon coconut oil

Tools/Equipment:

- Small saucepan
- Container for storage

Instructions:

1. Melt beeswax and coconut oil over low heat.
2. Add castor oil and stir until combined.
3. Pour into the container and let cool.

Application Tips:

- Rub a small amount between fingers and style as desired.

Storage and Shelf Life:

- Store at room temperature; lasts up to 3 months.

Safety Notes:

- Avoid contact with eyes.

With castor oil, you can enjoy a well-conditioned, itch-free beard that's naturally soft and healthy.

Post-Shave Skin Conditioning: Soothing Irritation and Hydrating Skin

Castor oil is an excellent option for post-shave skin care, thanks to its anti-inflammatory and deeply moisturizing properties. It helps to soothe irritation, reduce redness, and hydrate freshly shaved skin, providing relief from razor burn and leaving your skin smooth and comfortable.

How to Use Castor Oil After Shaving:

- **Apply to Damp Skin**: After shaving, lightly pat your skin dry and then massage a small amount of castor oil onto the skin. Damp skin helps the oil absorb more easily.
- **Combine with Calming Oils**: Mix castor oil with a few drops of chamomile or tea tree oil to create a soothing post-shave blend that can calm redness and reduce any discomfort.
- **Focus on Sensitive Areas**: Apply more to areas prone to razor burn or dryness to keep your skin moisturized and irritation-free.

Post-Shave Skin Soother for Redness and Irritation

Purpose/Benefits: Calms skin irritation and hydrates freshly shaved skin.

Ingredients:

- 1 tablespoon castor oil
- 2 drops tea tree oil
- 1 drop chamomile oil

Tools/Equipment:

- Small bottle

Instructions:

1. Mix all oils in the bottle and shake well.

Application Tips:

- Apply a few drops to damp skin after shaving.

Storage and Shelf Life:

- Store in a cool place; lasts up to 3 months.

Safety Notes:

- Perform a patch test first to ensure no sensitivity.

Anti-Itch Beard Balm for New Growth

Purpose/Benefits: Reduces itchiness and soothes skin during early beard growth.

Ingredients:

- 1 tablespoon castor oil
- 1 tablespoon shea butter
- 2 drops peppermint essential oil

Tools/Equipment:

- Mixing bowl
- Storage container

Instructions:

1. Blend castor oil, shea butter, and peppermint oil until smooth.
2. Store in a container.

Application Tips:

- Apply a small amount to the beard and massage in.

Storage and Shelf Life:

- Keep in a cool place; lasts up to 3 months.

Safety Notes:

- Avoid applying near eyes.

Hydrating Face Oil for Dry, Post-Shave Skin

Purpose/Benefits: Hydrates and soothes skin after shaving.

Ingredients:

- 1 tablespoon castor oil
- 1 tablespoon grapeseed oil
- 2 drops lavender essential oil

Tools/Equipment:

- Dropper bottle

Instructions:

1. Combine ingredients in the dropper bottle.

Application Tips:

- Apply to damp skin post-shave to lock in moisture.

Storage and Shelf Life:

- Store for up to 6 months.

Safety Notes:

- Patch test before full application.

DIY Beard Conditioning Balm for Daily Use

Purpose/Benefits: Tames unruly beard hair and locks in moisture.

Ingredients:

- 1 tablespoon castor oil
- 1 tablespoon beeswax
- 2 drops sandalwood essential oil

Tools/Equipment:

- Small saucepan
- Storage container

Instructions:

1. Melt beeswax, add castor oil, then mix in essential oil.
2. Pour into a container and let cool.

Application Tips:

- Apply daily to keep beard conditioned and soft.

Storage and Shelf Life:

- Store in a cool place; lasts up to 3 months.

Safety Notes:

- Keep away from eyes.

Castor Oil and Aloe Post-Shave Gel for Sensitive Skin

Purpose/Benefits: A cooling gel to soothe and hydrate skin after shaving.

Ingredients:

- 1 tablespoon castor oil
- 2 tablespoons aloe vera gel
- 2 drops chamomile essential oil

Tools/Equipment:

- Mixing bowl
- Small container

Instructions:

1. Mix castor oil and aloe vera gel until smooth.
2. Add chamomile oil and transfer to container.

Application Tips:

- Apply to freshly shaved skin.

Storage and Shelf Life:

- Store in the fridge; lasts up to 2 weeks.

Safety Notes:

- Avoid applying near eyes.

Natural Pomade with Castor Oil for Flexible Hold

Purpose/Benefits: Provides a soft hold for styling while conditioning hair.

Ingredients:

- 1 tablespoon castor oil
- 1 tablespoon shea butter
- 1 teaspoon beeswax

Tools/Equipment:

- Small saucepan
- Container for storage

Instructions:

1. Melt the shea butter and beeswax in a saucepan over low heat.
2. Stir in the castor oil until well-blended.
3. Pour into a container and let cool.

Application Tips:

- Use a small amount to style hair as desired, adding hold and shine.

Storage and Shelf Life:

- Store at room temperature; lasts up to 3 months.

Safety Notes:

- Avoid contact with eyes.

Castor Oil and Tea Tree Beard Cleanser for Acne-Prone Skin

Purpose/Benefits: Cleanses the beard and helps reduce acne in the beard area.

Ingredients:

- 1 tablespoon castor oil
- 1 tablespoon jojoba oil
- 3 drops tea tree essential oil

Tools/Equipment:

- Dropper bottle

Instructions:

1. Combine all oils in the dropper bottle and shake to mix.

Application Tips:

- Apply a few drops and massage into the beard area, then rinse thoroughly.

Storage and Shelf Life:

- Store in a cool, dark place; lasts up to 6 months.

Safety Notes:

- Perform a patch test to ensure no sensitivity.

Beard Thickening Oil Blend with Castor Oil and Eucalyptus

Purpose/Benefits: Helps create a fuller, healthier-looking beard.

Ingredients:

- 1 tablespoon castor oil
- 1 tablespoon coconut oil
- 2 drops eucalyptus essential oil

Tools/Equipment:

- Small bottle

Instructions:

2. Mix the oils in a bottle and shake to blend.

Application Tips:

- Massage a few drops into the beard daily.

Storage and Shelf Life:

- Store in a cool, dark place; lasts up to 6 months.

Safety Notes:

- Avoid direct contact with eyes.

By incorporating castor oil into your post-shave routine, you can keep your skin calm, hydrated, and protected from the effects of shaving.

DIY Grooming Blends: Beard Oils, Aftershave Balms, and Skin Soothers

Creating your own grooming blends with castor oil is simple and allows you to enjoy natural, chemical-free products tailored to your needs. Here are a few easy recipes to get you started:

Beard Thickening Oil Blend with Castor Oil and Eucalyptus

Purpose/Benefits: Helps create a fuller, healthier-looking beard.

Ingredients:

- 1 tablespoon castor oil
- 1 tablespoon coconut oil
- 2 drops eucalyptus essential oil

Tools/Equipment:

- Small bottle

Instructions:

3. Mix the oils in a bottle and shake to blend.

Application Tips:

- Massage a few drops into the beard daily.

Storage and Shelf Life:

- Store in a cool, dark place; lasts up to 6 months.

Safety Notes:

Avoid direct contact with eyes

Each blend is designed to enhance your grooming routine with natural ingredients, giving you effective results without additives or harsh chemicals.

Oral Health and Hygiene

Gum Health: Supporting Oral Health and Reducing Gum Inflammation

Castor oil's antibacterial and anti-inflammatory properties make it a gentle, natural choice for maintaining healthy gums and reducing inflammation. Its ability to fight bacteria helps prevent issues like gingivitis, while its soothing properties make it ideal for reducing gum sensitivity and irritation.

How to Use Castor Oil for Gum Health:

- **Apply Directly to Gums**: Place a drop or two of castor oil on a clean fingertip or cotton swab, and gently massage it into your gums. This can help soothe any discomfort and improve gum health over time.
- **Combine with Coconut Oil**: For added benefits, mix castor oil with coconut oil, which also has natural antibacterial properties. Use this blend for a gentle gum massage or as part of your daily oral care routine.

Castor Oil Gum Soother for Sensitive Gums

Purpose/Benefits: Soothes inflammation and reduces gum sensitivity.

Ingredients:

- 1 teaspoon castor oil (organic, cold-pressed)
- 1 drop clove essential oil

Tools/Equipment:

- Small dish
- Cotton swab

Instructions:

1. Mix castor oil and clove oil in a small dish.
2. Dip a cotton swab in the mixture and apply it gently to sensitive areas of the gums.

Application Tips:

- Use once daily or as needed.

Storage and Shelf Life:

- Store in a cool, dark place; lasts up to 1 month.

Safety Notes:

- Avoid swallowing. Perform a patch test before applying.

Castor Oil and Aloe Oral Gel for Canker Sores

Purpose/Benefits: Soothes canker sores and promotes healing.

Ingredients:

- 1 teaspoon castor oil
- 1 teaspoon aloe vera gel

Tools/Equipment:

- Small bowl
- Cotton swab

Instructions:

1. Mix castor oil with aloe vera gel.
2. Apply directly to canker sore with a cotton swab.

Application Tips:

- Apply 2-3 times daily until sore is gone.

Storage and Shelf Life:

- Store in a cool place; lasts up to 1 week.

Safety Notes:

- Avoid swallowing large amounts.

Anti-Inflammatory Gum Rub with Castor Oil and Turmeric

Purpose/Benefits: Reduces gum inflammation and fights bacteria.

Ingredients:

- 1 teaspoon castor oil
- 1/4 teaspoon turmeric powder

Tools/Equipment:

- Small bowl
- Cotton swab

Instructions:

1. Mix castor oil and turmeric in a small bowl.
2. Apply to gums using a cotton swab.

Application Tips:

- Use 1-2 times daily, especially around inflamed areas.

Storage and Shelf Life:

- Prepare fresh each use.

Safety Notes:

- Rinse mouth thoroughly after 5 minutes to prevent staining.

Castor Oil and Coconut Oil Pulling Solution for Detox

Purpose/Benefits: Detoxifies and improves overall oral health.

Ingredients:

- 1 tablespoon castor oil
- 1 tablespoon coconut oil

Tools/Equipment:

- Small cup

Instructions:

1. Mix castor oil and coconut oil in a small cup.
2. Swish in your mouth for 10-15 minutes, then spit out.

Application Tips:

- Perform daily for optimal results.

Storage and Shelf Life:

- Store at room temperature; lasts up to 1 month.

Safety Notes:

- Do not swallow.

Herbal Castor Oil Mouthwash for Gum Health

Purpose/Benefits: Supports gum health and a balanced oral microbiome.

Ingredients:

- 1 cup distilled water
- 1 teaspoon castor oil
- 1 drop rosemary essential oil
- 1 drop sage essential oil

Tools/Equipment:

- Small bottle with lid

Instructions:

1. Mix all ingredients in a small bottle and shake well.

Application Tips:

- Swish 1 tablespoon in mouth for 30 seconds, then spit.

Storage and Shelf Life:

- Store in a cool place; lasts up to 2 weeks.

Safety Notes:

- Do not swallow.

Toothache Relief Oil with Castor Oil and Clove

Purpose/Benefits: Temporarily relieves toothache pain.

Ingredients:

- 1 teaspoon castor oil
- 1 drop clove essential oil

Tools/Equipment:

- Cotton swab

Instructions:

1. Mix castor oil and clove oil.
2. Apply to the aching tooth with a cotton swab.

Application Tips:

- Use sparingly as needed.

Storage and Shelf Life:

- Store in a cool place; lasts up to 1 week.

Safety Notes:

- Avoid prolonged use without consulting a dentist.

Castor Oil and Eucalyptus Gum Stimulating Massage Oil

Purpose/Benefits: Stimulates gum circulation and supports health.

Ingredients:

- 1 teaspoon castor oil
- 1 drop eucalyptus essential oil

Tools/Equipment:

- Cotton swab

Instructions:

1. Mix castor oil and eucalyptus oil.
2. Massage gently onto gums with a cotton swab.

Application Tips:

- Use 1-2 times weekly for best results.

Storage and Shelf Life:

- Store in a cool place; lasts up to 1 month.

Safety Notes:

Avoid swallowing; do not use on children under 6.

Castor Oil Gum Healing Balm for Irritation and Swelling

Purpose/Benefits: Soothes and reduces gum irritation.

Ingredients:

- 1 teaspoon castor oil
- 1 drop chamomile essential oil

Tools/Equipment:

- Small bowl
- Cotton swab

Instructions:

1. Mix castor oil and chamomile oil in a bowl.
2. Apply with a cotton swab to affected gums.

Application Tips:

- Apply twice daily for best results.

Storage and Shelf Life:

- Store in a cool, dark place; lasts up to 1 month.

Safety Notes:

- Avoid swallowing. Test for sensitivity first.

Natural Mouthwash with Castor Oil for Fresh Breath

Purpose/Benefits: Freshens breath and supports oral hygiene without alcohol.

Ingredients:

- 1 cup distilled water
- 1 teaspoon castor oil
- 3 drops peppermint essential oil

Tools/Equipment:

- Small bottle with lid

Instructions:

1. Combine all ingredients in the bottle and shake well before each use.

Application Tips:

- Swish 1 tablespoon in your mouth for 30 seconds, then spit out.

Storage and Shelf Life:

- Store in a cool, dark place; lasts up to 2 weeks.

Safety Notes:

- Do not swallow.

Anti-Bacterial Mouth Rinse for Daily Oral Hygiene

Purpose/Benefits: Reduces bacteria and freshens breath.

Ingredients:

- 1 cup distilled water
- 1 teaspoon castor oil
- 1 drop tea tree essential oil

Tools/Equipment:

- Small bottle

Instructions:

1. Mix all ingredients in the bottle and shake well.

Application Tips:

- Swish 1 tablespoon in your mouth for 30 seconds, then spit out.

Storage and Shelf Life:

- Store in a cool place; lasts up to 2 weeks.

Safety Notes:

- Avoid swallowing. Not recommended for children.

Castor Oil and Salt Gargle for Sore Throat Relief

Purpose/Benefits: Soothes a sore throat and reduces inflammation.

Ingredients:

- 1 cup warm water
- 1/2 teaspoon castor oil
- 1/4 teaspoon salt

Tools/Equipment:

- Small glass

Instructions:

1. Combine ingredients in a glass, stirring until salt dissolves.

Application Tips:

- Gargle for 30 seconds, then spit out.

Storage and Shelf Life:

- Prepare fresh each time.

Safety Notes:

- Avoid swallowing.

Natural Castor Oil Teeth Whitener

Purpose/Benefits: Brightens teeth naturally without harsh chemicals.

Ingredients:

- 1 teaspoon castor oil
- 1/4 teaspoon hydrogen peroxide (3% solution)

Tools/Equipment:

- Small bowl

Instructions:

1. Mix castor oil and hydrogen peroxide.
2. Dip your toothbrush in the mixture and brush gently.

Application Tips:

- Use once a week to avoid overuse.

Storage and Shelf Life:

- Prepare fresh each use.

Safety Notes:

- Avoid swallowing and consult a dentist if you have sensitivity.

Castor Oil Tooth Powder for Plaque Removal

Purpose/Benefits: Helps remove plaque and support enamel health.

Ingredients:

- 1 tablespoon bentonite clay
- 1 tablespoon baking soda
- 1 teaspoon castor oil

Tools/Equipment:

- Small jar

Instructions:

1. Mix all ingredients in a jar until combined.

Application Tips:

- Dip a damp toothbrush into the powder and brush gently.

Storage and Shelf Life:

- Store in a cool, dry place; lasts up to 1 month.

Safety Notes:

- Use sparingly on sensitive teeth.

Castor Oil Lip Balm for Dry, Chapped Lips

Purpose/Benefits: Moisturizes and protects chapped lips.

Ingredients:

- 1 tablespoon castor oil
- 1 tablespoon beeswax pellets
- 1 teaspoon coconut oil

Tools/Equipment:

- Small heat-safe bowl
- Lip balm container

Instructions:

1. Melt beeswax and coconut oil in a heat-safe bowl over hot water.
2. Stir in castor oil until well mixed.
3. Pour the mixture into a container and allow it to cool.

Application Tips:

- Apply as needed for hydration.

Storage and Shelf Life:

- Store in a cool, dry place; lasts up to 3 months.

Safety Notes:

- Patch test if sensitive to beeswax.

Healing Cheek and Tongue Soother with Castor Oil

Purpose/Benefits: Eases irritation on the inner cheek or tongue from accidental bites.

Ingredients:

- 1 teaspoon castor oil
- 1/2 teaspoon calendula extract

Tools/Equipment:

- Cotton swab

Instructions:

1. Mix castor oil with calendula extract.
2. Use a cotton swab to apply gently to the irritated area.

Application Tips:

- Apply 2-3 times daily until healed.

Storage and Shelf Life:

- Store in a cool, dark place; lasts up to 2 weeks.

Safety Notes:

- Avoid swallowing.

Using castor oil regularly as part of your oral care can help maintain strong, healthy gums naturally.

Mouth Ulcer Treatment: Soothing and Healing Ulcers Naturally

If you struggle with mouth ulcers, castor oil can provide a natural way to relieve discomfort and support healing. Its anti-inflammatory and moisturizing qualities help reduce pain and promote faster recovery, offering a gentle alternative to medicated treatments.

How to Use Castor Oil for Mouth Ulcers:

- **Apply Directly to the Ulcer**: Using a clean cotton swab, dab a small amount of castor oil onto the ulcer. The oil will form a protective layer, helping to ease irritation and support healing.
- **Repeat as Needed**: For best results, reapply castor oil 2-3 times a day until the ulcer improves.

Castor Oil Treatment for Mouth Ulcers

Purpose/Benefits: Alleviates pain and supports healing.

Ingredients:

- 1 teaspoon castor oil
- 1/2 teaspoon aloe vera gel

Tools/Equipment:

- Cotton swab

Instructions:

1. Mix castor oil and aloe vera gel.
2. Apply directly to ulcers using a cotton swab.

Application Tips:

- Apply 2-3 times daily.

Storage and Shelf Life:

- Store in a cool place; lasts up to 1 week.

Safety Notes:

- Avoid swallowing.

Overnight Castor Oil Mouth Ulcer Relief Treatment

Purpose/Benefits: Provides nighttime relief for mouth ulcers.

Ingredients:

- 1 teaspoon castor oil
- 1 drop chamomile essential oil

Tools/Equipment:

- Cotton swab

Instructions:

1. Mix castor oil and chamomile oil.
2. Apply directly to the ulcer before bed with a cotton swab.

Application Tips:

- Use nightly until ulcer heals.

Storage and Shelf Life:

- Store in a cool place; lasts up to 1 week.

Safety Notes:

- Avoid swallowing.

This easy method allows you to treat mouth ulcers effectively with castor oil, reducing discomfort and encouraging a quicker recovery.

DIY Mouth Care Recipes: Castor Oil Mouthwashes and Oral Health Remedies

Creating your own natural mouth care products with castor oil is simple and offers a safe, chemical-free alternative to commercial oral health products. Here are a few easy recipes to try:

<u>DIY Minty Tooth Gel for Kids with Castor Oil</u>

Purpose/Benefits: Gently cleans children's teeth and freshens breath.

Ingredients:

- 1 teaspoon castor oil
- 1 teaspoon xylitol powder (optional, for sweetness)
- 1 drop peppermint essential oil

Tools/Equipment:

- Small container

Instructions:

1. Mix all ingredients in a small container until smooth.

Application Tips:

- Use a pea-sized amount for brushing, then rinse.

Storage and Shelf Life:

- Store in a cool place; lasts up to 2 weeks.

Safety Notes:

- Ensure kids do not swallow.

DIY Breath Freshening Spray with Castor Oil

Purpose/Benefits: Freshens breath on the go.

Ingredients:

- 1 tablespoon distilled water
- 1/2 teaspoon castor oil
- 2 drops peppermint essential oil

Tools/Equipment:

- Small spray bottle

Instructions:

1. Combine all ingredients in the spray bottle and shake well.

Application Tips:

- Spritz once in the mouth for fresh breath.

Storage and Shelf Life:

- Store in a cool place; lasts up to 2 weeks.

Safety Notes:

- Do not swallow large quantities.

DIY Toothpaste with Castor Oil and Baking Soda

Purpose/Benefits: Cleans teeth naturally and removes surface stains.

Ingredients:

- 1 tablespoon castor oil
- 1 tablespoon baking soda
- 1 teaspoon coconut oil

Tools/Equipment:

- Small jar

Instructions:

1. Mix all ingredients in the jar until smooth.

Application Tips:

- Use a small amount on your toothbrush, then rinse thoroughly.

Storage and Shelf Life:

- Store at room temperature; lasts up to 1 month.

Safety Notes:

- Do not use on highly sensitive teeth due to baking soda's abrasiveness.

Eco-Friendly Household and Pet Care Applications

Non-Toxic Cleaning Solutions: Antifungal and Antibacterial Uses for the Home

Castor oil's natural antifungal and antibacterial properties make it an ideal ingredient for creating safe, non-toxic cleaning solutions. Unlike chemical cleaners, castor oil-based cleaners offer a safer choice for households, especially those with children or pets, while still effectively disinfecting and cleaning.

Natural All-Purpose Cleaner with Castor Oil and Lemon

Purpose/Benefits: A versatile, all-purpose cleaner that safely cleans various surfaces with antibacterial properties.

Ingredients:

- 2 cups water
- 1 tablespoon castor oil
- 1/4 cup white vinegar
- 10 drops lemon essential oil

Tools/Equipment:

- Spray bottle
- Microfiber cloth

Instructions:

1. Combine water, castor oil, and vinegar in a spray bottle.
2. Add lemon essential oil, then shake well.

Application Tips:

- Spray on surfaces like countertops and tables, then wipe with a microfiber cloth.

Storage and Shelf Life:

- Store at room temperature; lasts up to 1 month.

Safety Notes:

- Avoid use on marble or granite due to vinegar content.

Castor Oil Glass and Mirror Cleaner

Purpose/Benefits: Leaves glass and mirrors streak-free and shiny without harsh chemicals.

Ingredients:

- 1 cup water
- 1 tablespoon castor oil
- 1/4 cup white vinegar

Tools/Equipment:

- Spray bottle
- Lint-free cloth

Instructions:

1. Mix water, castor oil, and vinegar in a spray bottle.
2. Shake well before each use.

Application Tips:

- Spray on glass and wipe clean with a lint-free cloth.

Storage and Shelf Life:

- Store at room temperature; lasts up to 1 month.

Safety Notes:

- Test on a small area if using on specialty glass.

Antibacterial Castor Oil Kitchen Degreaser

Purpose/Benefits: Cuts through grease and disinfects surfaces naturally.

Ingredients:

- 1 cup water
- 1 tablespoon castor oil
- 1/4 cup baking soda
- 5 drops tea tree essential oil

Tools/Equipment:

- Spray bottle
- Sponge

Instructions:

1. Combine water, castor oil, baking soda, and tea tree oil in a spray bottle.
2. Shake well before use.

Application Tips:

- Spray on greasy surfaces and scrub with a sponge.

Storage and Shelf Life:

- Store in a cool place; lasts up to 1 month.

Safety Notes:

- Avoid prolonged contact with aluminum surfaces.

DIY Castor Oil and Citrus Wood Polish

Purpose/Benefits: Brings out the natural shine in wood surfaces without chemicals.

Ingredients:

- 1/4 cup castor oil
- 1/4 cup olive oil
- 10 drops lemon essential oil

Tools/Equipment:

- Soft cloth

Instructions:

1. Mix castor oil, olive oil, and lemon essential oil in a small bowl.
2. Apply a small amount to a cloth and rub onto wood.

Application Tips:

- Use once a month to maintain wood polish and shine.

Storage and Shelf Life:

- Store in a cool place; lasts up to 3 months.

Safety Notes:

- Test on a small area of wood before full application.

Natural Bathroom Cleaner with Castor Oil and Tea Tree

Purpose/Benefits: Disinfects and cleans bathroom surfaces with antibacterial properties.

Ingredients:

- 2 cups water
- 1 tablespoon castor oil
- 1/4 cup vinegar
- 10 drops tea tree essential oil

Tools/Equipment:

- Spray bottle
- Scrub brush

Instructions:

1. Combine all ingredients in a spray bottle and shake well.

Application Tips:

- Spray on bathroom surfaces and scrub with a brush.

Storage and Shelf Life:

- Store at room temperature; lasts up to 1 month.

Safety Notes:

- Avoid using on marble due to vinegar content.

Eco-Friendly Floor Cleaner with Castor Oil and Essential Oils

Purpose/Benefits: Safely cleans and freshens floors with natural ingredients.

Ingredients:

- 1 gallon warm water
- 1 tablespoon castor oil
- 10 drops lavender essential oil
- 10 drops eucalyptus essential oil

Tools/Equipment:

- Mop or microfiber cloth

Instructions:

1. Mix all ingredients in a bucket of warm water.
2. Mop as usual.

Application Tips:

- Use once a week for clean, fresh-smelling floors.

Storage and Shelf Life:

- Prepare fresh for each use.

Safety Notes:

- Test on a small area if using on delicate floors.

DIY Castor Oil-Based Dish Soap

Purpose/Benefits: Cleans dishes without harsh chemicals, gentle on hands.

Ingredients:

- 1/2 cup castor oil
- 1/2 cup liquid Castile soap
- 10 drops lemon essential oil

Tools/Equipment:

- Squeeze bottle

Instructions:

1. Mix all ingredients in a squeeze bottle.
2. Shake gently to combine.

Application Tips:

- Use as regular dish soap.

Storage and Shelf Life:

- Store at room temperature; lasts up to 1 month.

Safety Notes:

- Avoid adding more castor oil to prevent greasiness.

Laundry Stain Remover with Castor Oil and Baking Soda

Purpose/Benefits: Lifts stains from fabrics naturally.

Ingredients:

- 1 tablespoon castor oil
- 2 tablespoons baking soda
- 1/4 cup water

Tools/Equipment:

- Small bowl

Instructions:

1. Mix castor oil and baking soda in water to create a paste.
2. Apply to stains and let sit for 15 minutes before washing.

Application Tips:

- Use as needed on stained areas before washing.

Storage and Shelf Life:

- Prepare fresh for each use.

Safety Notes:

- Test on a small area of fabric for colorfastness.

Non-Toxic Castor Oil Air Freshener Spray

Purpose/Benefits: Freshens up any room without artificial fragrances.

Ingredients:

- 1 cup water
- 1 tablespoon castor oil
- 10 drops peppermint essential oil
- 10 drops lemon essential oil

Tools/Equipment:

- Spray bottle

Instructions:

1. Combine all ingredients in a spray bottle and shake well.

Application Tips:

- Spray in any room for a quick refresh.

Storage and Shelf Life:

- Store at room temperature; lasts up to 1 month.

Safety Notes:

- Shake well before each use as ingredients may separate.

Castor Oil Mold and Mildew Remover

Purpose/Benefits: Cleans mold and mildew in damp areas like bathrooms.

Ingredients:

- 1 cup white vinegar
- 1 tablespoon castor oil
- 10 drops tea tree essential oil

Tools/Equipment:

- Spray bottle
- Scrub brush

Instructions:

1. Combine vinegar, castor oil, and tea tree oil in a spray bottle.
2. Shake well and spray on moldy areas.

Application Tips:

- Let sit for 10 minutes before scrubbing.

Storage and Shelf Life:

- Store in a cool place; lasts up to 1 month.

Safety Notes:

Wear gloves and ensure good ventilation when applying.

Pest Control: Natural Pest Deterrent for Gardens and Indoor Use

Castor oil can be an effective and eco-friendly solution for deterring common pests without harming your plants, pets, or environment. Its natural properties make it useful both indoors and in the garden, offering a safe alternative to chemical pesticides.

Natural Garden Pest Repellent with Castor Oil

Purpose/Benefits: A safe, effective spray to repel pests like aphids, ants, and mites in the garden.

Ingredients:

- 1 tablespoon castor oil
- 1 tablespoon garlic juice or crushed garlic
- 10 drops peppermint essential oil
- 2 cups water

Tools/Equipment:

- Spray bottle
- Strainer (if using crushed garlic)

Instructions:

1. Combine water, castor oil, garlic, and peppermint oil in a spray bottle.
2. Shake well to mix ingredients. If using crushed garlic, strain before pouring into the spray bottle.

Application Tips:

- Spray directly on plants every 5-7 days to deter pests.
- Reapply after rain.

Storage and Shelf Life:

- Store in a cool, dark place; lasts up to 2 weeks.

Safety Notes:

- Avoid spraying directly on edible parts of plants; wash before consumption.

Indoor Insect Repellent with Castor Oil and Eucalyptus

Purpose/Benefits: Keeps indoor areas free from insects using a natural, non-toxic formula.

Ingredients:

- 1 tablespoon castor oil
- 10 drops eucalyptus essential oil
- 1 cup water

Tools/Equipment:

- Spray bottle

Instructions:

1. Mix castor oil, eucalyptus oil, and water in a spray bottle.
2. Shake well before each use.

Application Tips:

- Spray around windows, doors, and baseboards to keep bugs away.
- Reapply weekly or as needed.

Storage and Shelf Life:

- Store in a cool, dark place; lasts up to 1 month.

Safety Notes:

- Avoid spraying directly on pets or near their bedding.

Castor Oil Ant Barrier for Home Perimeters

Purpose/Benefits: Creates a natural ant barrier to prevent ants from entering the home.

Ingredients:

- 1 tablespoon castor oil
- 10 drops clove essential oil
- 1 cup water

Tools/Equipment:

- Spray bottle
- Soft cloth or brush (for applying around small areas)

Instructions:

1. Combine castor oil, clove oil, and water in a spray bottle.
2. Shake well to mix.

Application Tips:

- Spray along baseboards, window sills, and door frames.
- Use a soft cloth or brush to apply in smaller spaces.

Storage and Shelf Life:

- Store at room temperature; lasts up to 1 month.

Safety Notes:

- Avoid areas accessible to pets and children, as clove oil can be strong.

Pet-Safe Flea Spray with Castor Oil and Neem

Purpose/Benefits: A flea-repellent spray that's safe for pets and effective for deterring fleas.

Ingredients:

- 1 tablespoon castor oil
- 1 tablespoon neem oil
- 2 cups water

Tools/Equipment:

- Spray bottle

Instructions:

1. Mix castor oil, neem oil, and water in a spray bottle.
2. Shake well before each use.

Application Tips:

- Lightly mist pet bedding and areas where pets frequently rest.
- Reapply weekly or after washing pet bedding.

Storage and Shelf Life:

- Store in a cool, dark place; lasts up to 1 month.

Safety Notes:

- Do not spray directly on pets; use only in their living spaces.

Rodent Deterrent Spray with Castor Oil and Peppermint

Purpose/Benefits: A natural rodent-repellent spray that is safe for homes with pets.

Ingredients:

- 1 tablespoon castor oil
- 10 drops peppermint essential oil
- 1 cup water

Tools/Equipment:

- Spray bottle

Instructions:

1. Combine castor oil, peppermint oil, and water in a spray bottle.
2. Shake well before each use.

Application Tips:

- Spray around entry points, kitchen areas, and garage spaces.

- Reapply every 1-2 weeks or as needed.

Storage and Shelf Life:

- Store in a cool place; lasts up to 1 month.

Safety Notes:

- Avoid spraying directly onto surfaces that pets may lick or chew.

Furniture and Wood Care

DIY Castor Oil Furniture Polish for Wood Conditioning

Purpose/Benefits: A nourishing polish that enhances shine and protects wooden surfaces naturally.

Ingredients:

- 2 tablespoons castor oil
- 1 tablespoon beeswax pellets
- 1 tablespoon olive oil (optional for added shine)

Tools/Equipment:

- Small saucepan
- Soft cloth

Instructions:

1. Melt the beeswax in a small saucepan over low heat.
2. Remove from heat, add castor oil (and olive oil, if using), and stir until well combined.
3. Allow the mixture to cool slightly before applying.

Application Tips:

- Apply a small amount to a soft cloth and rub onto wooden surfaces in a circular motion.
- Buff with a clean cloth to enhance shine.

Storage and Shelf Life:

- Store in an airtight container; lasts up to 6 months.

Safety Notes:

- Test on a small, inconspicuous area first to ensure compatibility with the wood finish.

Leather Cleaner and Conditioner with Castor Oil

Purpose/Benefits: Cleans, softens, and conditions leather items, leaving them supple and protected.

Ingredients:

- 1 tablespoon castor oil
- 1 tablespoon olive oil

Tools/Equipment:

- Soft cloth

Instructions:

1. Combine castor oil and olive oil in a small container.
2. Dip a soft cloth into the oil mixture and gently rub onto the leather surface.

Application Tips:

- Use sparingly and rub in a circular motion for even application.
- Buff with a clean cloth to remove any excess oil.

Storage and Shelf Life:

- Store mixture in a cool, dark place; lasts up to 3 months.

Safety Notes:

- Test on a small area first, especially on delicate or light-colored leather.

Castor Oil Scratch Remover for Wooden Surfaces

Purpose/Benefits: Helps reduce the appearance of scratches on wooden furniture, restoring a smooth look.

Ingredients:

- 1 tablespoon castor oil
- 1 tablespoon walnut oil (or olive oil)

Tools/Equipment:

- Soft cloth

Instructions:

1. Mix castor oil and walnut oil in a small bowl.
2. Dip a soft cloth into the mixture and rub over the scratch in a circular motion.

Application Tips:

- Let the oil sit for 10-15 minutes, then buff the area with a clean cloth.

Storage and Shelf Life:

- Prepare fresh as needed.

Safety Notes:

- Suitable for darker woods, as walnut oil may slightly darken light wood.

Natural Upholstery Cleaner with Castor Oil and Vinegar

Purpose/Benefits: A gentle cleaner designed to freshen and clean upholstery safely.

Ingredients:

- 1 tablespoon castor oil
- 2 tablespoons white vinegar
- 10 drops lemon essential oil (optional for fragrance)
- 1 cup water

Tools/Equipment:

- Spray bottle
- Soft cloth or sponge

Instructions:

1. Combine castor oil, vinegar, essential oil, and water in a spray bottle.
2. Shake well before each use.

Application Tips:

- Lightly spray onto upholstery and use a soft cloth or sponge to blot and clean.
- Avoid oversaturating fabric; always test on a small area first.

Storage and Shelf Life:

- Store in a cool, dark place; lasts up to 2 weeks.

Safety Notes:

- Not suitable for delicate or untreated fabrics.

Castor Oil-Based Metal Polish for Silver and Brass

Purpose/Benefits: A natural polish that restores shine to silver and brass without harsh chemicals.

Ingredients:

- 1 tablespoon castor oil
- 1 tablespoon baking soda
- 1 teaspoon white vinegar (for extra tarnish removal)

Tools/Equipment:

- Soft cloth

Instructions:

1. Combine castor oil, baking soda, and vinegar in a small bowl to form a paste.
2. Apply a small amount of the paste to a soft cloth and rub onto the metal surface in a circular motion.

Application Tips:

- Buff with a clean cloth after polishing to remove any residue and enhance shine.

Storage and Shelf Life:

- Prepare fresh as needed.

Safety Notes:

- Test on a small area first, as vinegar may react with certain metal finishes.

Pet Health: Safe Skin and Joint Remedies for Pets, Digestive Health Support

Castor oil can be beneficial for pets when used carefully. It is particularly helpful for soothing skin irritations, providing relief for joint discomfort, and supporting digestive health in moderation.

Castor Oil Paw Balm for Pets

Purpose/Benefits: A soothing balm to protect and moisturize pets' paw pads from rough surfaces and extreme weather conditions.

Ingredients:

- 1 tablespoon castor oil
- 1 tablespoon coconut oil
- 1 tablespoon beeswax (optional for extra protection)

Tools/Equipment:

- Small saucepan
- Spoon
- Small storage container

Instructions:

1. Melt the beeswax and coconut oil in a small saucepan over low heat.
2. Remove from heat, add castor oil, and stir until combined.
3. Pour into a small container and let it cool completely before use.

Application Tips:

- Apply a small amount to each paw pad, rubbing in gently.
- Use as needed, especially before walks on hot pavement or in cold weather.

Storage and Shelf Life:

- Store in a cool, dry place; lasts up to 6 months.

Safety Notes:

- Ensure pets do not lick excessively after application.

Natural Ear Cleaner for Pets with Castor Oil and Lavender

Purpose/Benefits: A gentle ear-cleaning solution to keep pet ears clean and reduce irritation.

Ingredients:

- 1 tablespoon castor oil
- 1 drop lavender essential oil
- 1/4 cup warm water

Tools/Equipment:

- Dropper or small bottle
- Cotton balls

Instructions:

1. Mix castor oil, lavender oil, and warm water in a small bottle.
2. Shake well before each use.

Application Tips:

- Dampen a cotton ball with the solution and gently wipe the inside of the pet's ears.
- Use once a week or as needed.

Storage and Shelf Life:

- Store in a cool place, away from direct sunlight; lasts up to 2 weeks.

Safety Notes:

- Avoid deep insertion into the ear canal. Consult a vet if there are signs of infection.

Castor Oil Coat Conditioner for Shiny Fur

Purpose/Benefits: A light conditioner for pets' coats, promoting a shiny, healthy appearance.

Ingredients:

- 1 tablespoon castor oil
- 1 tablespoon rosemary-infused water (optional for scent)

Tools/Equipment:

- Spray bottle

Instructions:

1. Mix castor oil and rosemary-infused water in a spray bottle.
2. Shake well before each use.

Application Tips:

- Lightly spray onto pet's coat and brush through to distribute evenly.
- Use once a week for best results.

Storage and Shelf Life:

- Store in a cool, dry place; lasts up to 1 month.

Safety Notes:

- Avoid contact with eyes and keep away from sensitive areas.

Pet-Friendly Castor Oil Hot Spot Soother

Purpose/Benefits: A soothing balm to ease itching and promote healing on hot spots.

Ingredients:

- 1 tablespoon castor oil
- 1 teaspoon aloe vera gel

Tools/Equipment:

- Small bowl

Instructions:

1. Mix castor oil and aloe vera gel in a small bowl until well combined.

Application Tips:

- Apply a thin layer directly to the affected area, avoiding excessive licking.
- Use once or twice daily until the hot spot improves.

Storage and Shelf Life:

- Store in the refrigerator; lasts up to 1 week.

Safety Notes:

- Consult a vet if the hot spot persists or worsens.

Pet Joint Relief Rub with Castor Oil and Turmeric

Purpose/Benefits: A gentle, soothing rub for pets experiencing joint discomfort.

Ingredients:

- 1 tablespoon castor oil
- 1/4 teaspoon turmeric powder

Tools/Equipment:

- Small bowl

Instructions:

1. Mix castor oil and turmeric powder until smooth.

Application Tips:

- Gently massage onto the affected joint once daily.
- Avoid areas pets can easily lick.

Storage and Shelf Life:

- Store in a cool, dry place; lasts up to 1 week.

Safety Notes:

- Test a small area for sensitivity before applying to larger areas.

Natural Digestive Aid for Pets with Castor Oil (Vet Consult Recommended)

Purpose/Benefits: A gentle digestive aid to ease occasional constipation.

Ingredients:

- 1/8 teaspoon castor oil (for small pets, adjust amount based on size)

Tools/Equipment:

- Dropper

Instructions:

1. Measure the appropriate amount of castor oil based on pet size.

Application Tips:

- Administer by placing a drop on pet food once a week as needed.

- Always consult a veterinarian before use.

Storage and Shelf Life:

- Store castor oil in a cool, dark place; shelf life varies by bottle expiration.

Safety Notes:

- Avoid use in young, elderly, or chronically ill pets without vet guidance.

Castor Oil Pet Grooming Spray for Flea and Tick Prevention

Purpose/Benefits: A pet-friendly grooming spray to help repel fleas and ticks while nourishing fur.

Ingredients:

- 1 tablespoon castor oil
- 5 drops neem oil (flea repellent)
- 1 cup water

Tools/Equipment:

- Spray bottle

Instructions:

1. Mix castor oil, neem oil, and water in a spray bottle.
2. Shake well before each use.

Application Tips:

- Lightly mist onto pet's coat, avoiding face and sensitive areas.
- Use once a week or before outdoor activities.

Storage and Shelf Life:

- Store in a cool place, away from sunlight; lasts up to 1 month.

Safety Notes:

- Consult a veterinarian before use if your pet has sensitive skin.

Eco-Friendly Uses of Castor Oil

Soap Making

Moisturizing Castor Oil Soap Base

Purpose/Benefits: A gentle, moisturizing soap base made from castor oil, coconut oil, and olive oil, known for creating a rich lather that cleanses without stripping skin.

Ingredients:

- 1 cup castor oil
- 1 cup coconut oil
- 1 cup olive oil
- 4 oz lye (sodium hydroxide)
- 10 oz distilled water

Tools/Equipment:

- Heatproof container for mixing lye
- Mixing spoon
- Soap mold
- Thermometer

Instructions:

1. In a heatproof container, slowly add lye to distilled water (never add water to lye) and let it cool to 110°F.
2. In a separate pot, combine castor oil, coconut oil, and olive oil, heating to 110°F.
3. Combine the lye water with the oil mixture, blending until you achieve a "trace" consistency.
4. Pour into soap mold and let it set for 24 hours before unmolding.
5. Cure the bars in a cool, dry place for 4-6 weeks.

Application Tips:

- Use as a base for adding fragrances, colorants, or other ingredients for personalized soap bars.

Storage and Shelf Life:

- Store in a cool, dry place. Shelf life is approximately 1 year.

Safety Notes:

- Wear gloves and eye protection when working with lye.
- Ensure the soap fully cures before using to avoid skin irritation.

Castor Oil and Shea Butter Soap for Sensitive Skin

Purpose/Benefits: A hydrating soap made with castor oil and shea butter, designed for sensitive skin and offering a gentle, nourishing cleanse.

Ingredients:

- 1 cup castor oil
- 1/2 cup shea butter
- 1/2 cup olive oil
- 4 oz lye
- 10 oz distilled water

Tools/Equipment:

- Heatproof mixing container
- Soap mold
- Stick blender

Instructions:

1. Dissolve lye in distilled water and cool to 110°F.
2. Melt shea butter and combine with castor oil and olive oil at 110°F.
3. Blend oils and lye water together until trace forms.
4. Pour into mold, let set for 24 hours, and cure for 4-6 weeks.

Application Tips:

- Ideal for daily use on sensitive or dry skin.

Storage and Shelf Life:

- Keep bars dry between uses for longer life; shelf life is 1 year.

Safety Notes:

- Avoid contact with eyes and wear protective gear when handling lye.

Eco-Friendly Exfoliating Soap with Castor Oil and Coffee Grounds

Purpose/Benefits: An exfoliating soap that uses castor oil and coffee grounds to provide a deep cleanse and gentle exfoliation, ideal for rough or dry skin.

Ingredients:

- 1 cup castor oil
- 1 cup coconut oil
- 4 oz lye
- 10 oz distilled water
- 1/4 cup coffee grounds (used and dried)

Tools/Equipment:

- Mixing bowl
- Soap mold
- Spatula

Instructions:

1. Mix lye with water and cool to 110°F.
2. Heat castor and coconut oils to 110°F.
3. Blend lye solution with oils until trace forms, then mix in coffee grounds.
4. Pour into molds and cure for 4-6 weeks.

Application Tips:

- Use as an exfoliating soap 1-2 times a week.

Storage and Shelf Life:

- Store in a dry place; lasts up to 1 year.

Safety Notes:

- Avoid use on sensitive or broken skin.

Lavender Castor Oil Soap for Relaxing Aromatherapy

Purpose/Benefits: A calming lavender-scented soap with castor oil, ideal for evening baths to promote relaxation and reduce stress.

Ingredients:

- 1 cup castor oil
- 1 cup olive oil
- 4 oz lye
- 10 oz distilled water
- 10 drops lavender essential oil

Tools/Equipment:

- Heatproof container
- Soap mold
- Mixing spoon

Instructions:

1. Mix lye with water, allowing it to cool to 110°F.
2. Warm castor and olive oils to 110°F.
3. Blend lye solution with oils, and at trace, add lavender essential oil.
4. Pour into molds and let cure for 4-6 weeks.

Application Tips:

- Best used during evening baths or showers for a calming effect.

Storage and Shelf Life:

- Shelf life of 1 year, keep in a cool, dry place.

Safety Notes:

- Patch test before use if prone to skin sensitivity with essential oils.

Antibacterial Castor Oil Soap with Tea Tree Oil

Purpose/Benefits: A cleansing soap with castor oil and tea tree oil, suitable for acne-prone skin due to its antibacterial and anti-inflammatory properties.

Ingredients:

- 1 cup castor oil
- 1 cup coconut oil
- 4 oz lye
- 10 oz distilled water
- 5 drops tea tree essential oil

Tools/Equipment:

- Mixing container
- Soap mold
- Stick blender

Instructions:

1. Prepare lye water and cool to 110°F.
2. Heat castor and coconut oils to 110°F.
3. Blend lye solution with oils; add tea tree oil at trace.
4. Pour into molds, let set, and cure for 4-6 weeks.

Application Tips:

- Use as a facial or body soap for acne-prone skin.

Storage and Shelf Life:

- Store in a dry place; lasts 1 year.

Safety Notes:

- Perform a patch test for tea tree oil sensitivity.

Candle Making

Castor Oil and Soy Wax Candle for Clean Burning

Purpose/Benefits: A clean-burning, eco-friendly candle made from castor oil and soy wax, offering a sustainable alternative to paraffin candles.

Ingredients:

- 1 cup soy wax flakes
- 2 tbsp castor oil
- Cotton or wooden wick
- Candle container or mold

Tools/Equipment:

- Double boiler or heatproof bowl
- Stirring spoon
- Thermometer

Instructions:

1. Melt soy wax in a double boiler until fully liquid.
2. Stir in castor oil and heat until the mixture reaches about 140°F.
3. Place the wick in the container and pour the melted wax and oil mixture into it.
4. Allow the candle to cool and solidify for several hours before trimming the wick to 1/4 inch.

Application Tips:

- Light the candle and enjoy a clean-burning experience without soot or toxins.

Storage and Shelf Life:

- Store in a cool, dry place. Shelf life is around 1 year if kept away from heat and direct sunlight.

Safety Notes:

- Never leave a burning candle unattended.

Eco-Friendly Aromatherapy Candle with Castor Oil and Essential Oils

Purpose/Benefits: A scented candle made with castor oil, soy wax, and essential oils to create a calming, aromatic environment naturally.

Ingredients:

- 1 cup soy wax flakes
- 2 tbsp castor oil
- 20 drops essential oil (eucalyptus, citrus, or your choice)
- Cotton or wooden wick
- Candle container

Tools/Equipment:

- Double boiler or heatproof bowl
- Stirring spoon
- Thermometer

Instructions:

1. Melt soy wax in a double boiler, heating to about 140°F.
2. Stir in castor oil and essential oil of choice.
3. Place the wick in the container and pour the melted mixture in.
4. Allow the candle to cool and set before trimming the wick.

Application Tips:

- Use in living spaces or bedrooms to enjoy the aromatherapeutic benefits.

Storage and Shelf Life:

- Keep in a cool, dark place; lasts up to 1 year.

Safety Notes:

- Ensure the candle is in a stable container before lighting.

Lavender Castor Oil Candle for Relaxation

Purpose/Benefits: A relaxing candle made with castor oil, beeswax, and lavender essential oil to create a tranquil, stress-relieving atmosphere.

Ingredients:

- 1 cup beeswax
- 2 tbsp castor oil
- 15 drops lavender essential oil
- Cotton or wooden wick
- Candle container

Tools/Equipment:

- Double boiler or heatproof bowl
- Stirring spoon

Instructions:

1. Melt beeswax in a double boiler until fully liquid.
2. Stir in castor oil and lavender essential oil.
3. Place the wick in the container and pour in the wax mixture.
4. Allow the candle to cool and set completely.

Application Tips:

- Light this candle in the evening to promote relaxation and reduce stress.

Storage and Shelf Life:

- Store in a cool place; lasts up to 1 year.

Safety Notes:

- Keep out of reach of children and pets.

Unscented Castor Oil Emergency Candle

Purpose/Benefits: An unscented emergency candle with castor oil and soy wax, ideal as a backup lighting source.

Ingredients:

- 1 cup soy wax flakes
- 2 tbsp castor oil
- Cotton or wooden wick
- Candle container

Tools/Equipment:

- Double boiler or heatproof bowl
- Thermometer
- Stirring spoon

Instructions:

1. Melt soy wax in a double boiler.
2. Add castor oil and stir until fully combined.
3. Place the wick in the container, then pour in the melted wax mixture.
4. Let cool and solidify before trimming the wick.

Application Tips:

- Light during power outages or emergencies for a steady, long-lasting light source.

Storage and Shelf Life:

- Store in a cool, dry place; lasts indefinitely if stored well.

Safety Notes:

- Do not leave burning candles unattended.

Citronella Castor Oil Outdoor Candle for Mosquito Repellent

Purpose/Benefits: An outdoor candle with castor oil and citronella, perfect for repelling mosquitoes during outdoor gatherings.

Ingredients:

- 1 cup soy wax or beeswax
- 2 tbsp castor oil
- 20 drops citronella essential oil
- Cotton or wooden wick
- Outdoor candle container (metal or glass)

Tools/Equipment:

- Double boiler or heatproof bowl
- Stirring spoon
- Thermometer

Instructions:

1. Melt the wax in a double boiler and add castor oil.
2. Remove from heat and stir in citronella essential oil.
3. Place the wick in the container, pour the melted wax mixture over it, and let it cool to set.

Application Tips:

- Place the candle on outdoor tables to help repel mosquitoes naturally.

Storage and Shelf Life:

- Keep stored in a cool place when not in use. Shelf life is approximately 1 year.

- Use outdoors only, and do not leave unattended when lit.

Safety Notes:

Castor Oil Packs and Their Benefits

What Are Castor Oil Packs and How Do They Work?

Castor oil packs are a therapeutic, time-honored way of applying castor oil to specific areas of the body for targeted wellness benefits. In traditional natural medicine, these packs are used to deliver the healing properties of castor oil deeply into the body through a cloth application, often accompanied by gentle heat.

When you apply a castor oil pack, the oil penetrates the skin and helps stimulate circulation, reduce inflammation, and support the body's detoxification process. Castor oil packs work by enhancing lymphatic drainage, which aids in removing toxins and boosting immune function. Additionally, the warmth and rich texture of castor oil create a soothing experience, making it a wonderful tool for relaxation.

Common uses of castor oil packs include easing joint and muscle pain, supporting digestive health, and promoting overall relaxation. This simple, natural therapy is incredibly versatile and can be used for a range of wellness purposes.

Step-by-Step Guide to Making and Using Castor Oil Packs

Here's a step-by-step guide for creating and using a castor oil pack. This beginner-friendly process will guide you through the materials and application for a safe, effective experience.

Materials Needed:

- Organic, cold-pressed castor oil
- A piece of soft, clean cloth (flannel or cotton works best)
- Plastic wrap or a plastic sheet (to avoid staining)
- A heating pad or hot water bottle
- A towel (for extra warmth and protection)

Preparation and Application Steps:

1. **Prepare the Area:** Choose a comfortable, quiet spot where you can lie down for the duration of the treatment, as this process typically lasts 30–45 minutes.
2. **Soak the Cloth:** Pour a small amount of castor oil onto the cloth, enough to moisten it but not soak it excessively.
3. **Apply the Cloth:** Place the oil-soaked cloth on the target area of your body. Common placements include the abdomen (for digestive support), lower back (for pain relief), or over joints.
4. **Cover with Plastic:** Place a layer of plastic wrap or a plastic sheet over the cloth. This helps retain the heat and keeps the oil from staining surrounding surfaces.

5. **Add Heat**: Place a heating pad or hot water bottle over the plastic wrap. The heat enhances the oil's absorption and increases circulation in the area.
6. **Relax and Let It Work**: Lie down and relax for 30–45 minutes, allowing the castor oil pack to work its magic.
7. **Clean Up**: When finished, remove the pack and clean the area with a mild soap if needed. Store the cloth in a sealed bag for reuse (it can be used multiple times if properly stored).

Suggested Frequency:

- For general wellness, use castor oil packs 1–2 times per week.
- For specific health goals, such as joint pain or digestive support, increase frequency as comfortable, consulting a healthcare provider if needed.

Benefits for Pain Relief, Detox, and Relaxation

Castor oil packs provide a natural, effective way to support your body's wellness goals. Here are the primary benefits:

1. **Pain Relief**: Castor oil's anti-inflammatory properties make it ideal for soothing joint and muscle pain. When used as a pack, the oil penetrates deeply, helping to relieve tension and inflammation, particularly beneficial for arthritis and sore muscles.
2. **Detoxification**: Castor oil packs aid in lymphatic drainage, supporting your body's natural detoxification process. By promoting lymph flow, castor oil packs assist in eliminating toxins, enhancing liver health, and boosting immune function.
3. **Relaxation**: The warmth of a castor oil pack combined with its rich, moisturizing feel creates a calming, grounding experience. Many people use castor oil packs to reduce stress and enhance relaxation, especially at the end of a long day.

These benefits are supported by simple science: castor oil's ricinoleic acid promotes circulation and reduces inflammation, making it a gentle yet powerful option for holistic wellness.

Personal Story with Castor Oil Packs (Optional Inspiration)

For many people, castor oil packs have become a cherished part of their wellness routines. Here's a personal story that captures the simple yet profound benefits of this natural therapy:

"After a stressful week, I decided to try a castor oil pack for the first time. Placing it on my abdomen, I relaxed with a warm compress, letting the oil absorb. Within minutes, I felt the gentle warmth spreading, easing my tension. I repeated the process weekly and found it not only helped relieve occasional back pain but also supported my digestion, leaving me feeling lighter and more at ease. This simple ritual has become my go-to for unwinding and restoring balance."

Stories like this show how easy and accessible castor oil packs can be for anyone looking to support their body's natural wellness.

Final Thoughts: Your Journey with Castor Oil

Embracing the Natural Path to Health and Beauty

Reflect on the transformative power of castor oil and its ability to support your health and beauty naturally, without relying on harsh chemicals or complex routines. Embrace a simpler, more natural approach to self-care, knowing that castor oil offers a wide range of benefits for your wellness journey. By choosing castor oil, you're taking a step toward a holistic lifestyle that prioritizes your well-being and respects nature.

Inspiration for Continued Self-Care and Holistic Living

Let castor oil be your starting point for a balanced, nurturing routine that aligns with your health and wellness goals. Explore new ways to integrate castor oil into daily rituals, or try other natural remedies alongside it to enhance your self-care practice. Remember, small, consistent steps can lead to lasting changes in health and well-being. Celebrate the journey you've started, and continue to nurture yourself with confidence and curiosity.

Appendices

Appendix 1: List of Ingredients Used Across Recipes

This appendix provides a comprehensive, alphabetized list of ingredients mentioned throughout the book's recipes. Each ingredient includes a brief description and relevant benefits, helping you understand the purpose of each component in castor oil applications.

Aloe Vera Gel

- **Description**: A soothing gel extracted from the aloe vera plant.
- **Benefits**: Hydrates and soothes irritated skin, often used for burns, cuts, and as a natural moisturizer.

Beeswax

- **Description**: A natural wax produced by honey bees.
- **Benefits**: Acts as a barrier to lock in moisture, commonly used in balms and salves for its protective and hydrating properties.

Castor Oil

- **Description**: A thick, nutrient-rich oil from castor beans, rich in ricinoleic acid.
- **Benefits**: Known for its moisturizing, anti-inflammatory, and antibacterial properties; ideal for skin, hair, and joint health.

Coconut Oil

- **Description**: An edible oil extracted from coconut meat.
- **Benefits**: Provides deep hydration and has antibacterial properties, often combined with castor oil in skin and hair treatments.

Eucalyptus Essential Oil

- **Description**: An essential oil with a fresh, medicinal scent, derived from eucalyptus leaves.
- **Benefits**: Known for its antimicrobial and anti-inflammatory effects, used in respiratory and muscle relief blends.

Frankincense Essential Oil

- **Description**: A resin-derived essential oil with a warm, earthy aroma.
- **Benefits**: Promotes skin health and reduces the appearance of scars and wrinkles; calming and grounding for relaxation.

Jojoba Oil

- **Description**: A lightweight oil derived from the jojoba plant, similar to natural skin oils.
- **Benefits**: Moisturizes without clogging pores, making it suitable for all skin types, including acne-prone skin.

Lavender Essential Oil

- **Description**: A popular essential oil with a calming floral scent.
- **Benefits**: Soothes irritation, reduces anxiety, and promotes relaxation; commonly used in sleep aids and skin care.

Lemon Essential Oil

- **Description**: A bright, citrusy essential oil derived from lemon peels.
- **Benefits**: Known for its antibacterial and cleansing properties; used in cleaning products and skin care for brightening effects.

Olive Oil

- **Description**: A nourishing oil extracted from olives.
- **Benefits**: Moisturizes and soothes skin; rich in antioxidants and commonly used as a carrier oil in DIY recipes.

Peppermint Essential Oil

- **Description**: A refreshing essential oil with a cool, minty aroma.
- **Benefits**: Invigorates and soothes muscle pain; also used in hair treatments to stimulate circulation and promote growth.

Rosehip Oil

- **Description**: A rejuvenating oil derived from the seeds of wild rose bushes.
- **Benefits**: Known for its skin-repairing properties, helping to reduce scars, wrinkles, and hyperpigmentation.

Tea Tree Essential Oil

- **Description**: A potent essential oil with a medicinal scent, extracted from tea tree leaves.
- **Benefits**: Antibacterial, antifungal, and anti-inflammatory, commonly used for acne, dandruff, and minor cuts.

Vitamin E Oil

- **Description**: A nutrient-rich oil containing antioxidants.
- **Benefits**: Promotes skin healing and reduces signs of aging, often added to oil blends to extend shelf life.

Appendix 2: Glossary of Key Terms and Concepts

This glossary includes key terms and concepts that appear throughout the book. Each term is explained in simple, easy-to-understand language to support your journey with castor oil and natural wellness.

- **Antifungal**: A substance that helps prevent or stop the growth of fungi. Castor oil's antifungal properties make it useful for addressing conditions like dandruff and athlete's foot.
- **Antimicrobial**: A property that allows a substance to inhibit the growth of microorganisms, including bacteria, viruses, and fungi. Castor oil is antimicrobial, making it beneficial for skin care and minor wound treatment.
- **Antioxidant**: Compounds that help prevent or slow damage to cells caused by free radicals, which are unstable molecules. The antioxidants in castor oil, such as vitamin E, contribute to its anti-aging benefits.
- **Ayurveda**: A traditional system of medicine originating from India that focuses on balancing the body's energies (doshas) through natural treatments. Castor oil is often used in Ayurveda for its detoxifying and balancing effects.
- **Carrier Oil**: A base oil used to dilute essential oils for safe application on the skin. Castor oil is often used as a carrier oil, especially in blends for hair, skin, and wellness applications.
- **Cold-Pressed**: A method of extracting oil from seeds or plants without using heat, preserving more of the oil's natural nutrients. Cold-pressed castor oil retains higher levels of beneficial compounds.
- **Detoxification**: The process of removing toxins from the body. Castor oil is traditionally used to support detoxification, often through the use of castor oil packs applied to the abdomen.
- **Dosha**: In Ayurveda, doshas are the body's three energies—Vata, Pitta, and Kapha—that govern physical and mental processes. Castor oil is believed to balance doshas, particularly Pitta, due to its cooling and soothing properties.
- **Emollient**: A substance that softens and moisturizes the skin. Castor oil acts as an emollient, making it an effective ingredient in creams, balms, and moisturizers.
- **Essential Oil**: Concentrated plant extracts that capture the plant's natural scent and beneficial properties. Essential oils are often blended with castor oil for therapeutic applications like massage and aromatherapy.
- **Free Radicals**: Unstable molecules that can damage cells, contributing to aging and various diseases. Antioxidants in castor oil help neutralize free radicals, promoting skin health.
- **Lymphatic Drainage**: A process that encourages the movement of lymph fluid throughout the body to remove waste and toxins. Castor oil packs are thought to support lymphatic drainage.
- **Moisturizing**: The process of hydrating and protecting the skin. Castor oil's high fatty acid content makes it an excellent moisturizer, suitable for dry skin and hair.
- **Ricinoleic Acid**: A unique fatty acid found in high concentrations in castor oil, known for its anti-inflammatory, antibacterial, and moisturizing properties. Ricinoleic acid is responsible for many of castor oil's health and beauty benefits.
- **Saponification**: The chemical reaction that occurs when fats or oils mix with an alkali, producing soap. Castor oil is commonly used in soap making due to its lathering properties.
- **Topical Application**: Applying a substance directly to the skin. Castor oil is commonly used topically for skin, hair, and wellness benefits.
- **Transdermal**: A method of delivering active ingredients through the skin and into the bloodstream. Castor oil's penetrative qualities allow it to be used in transdermal applications, such as castor oil packs.
- **Toxin**: Harmful substances that can accumulate in the body, sometimes causing health issues. Castor oil is believed to aid in the removal of toxins, especially when used in detox practices like castor oil packs.

Exclusive Bonus: Unlock the Secrets of Castor Oil with Our Video Masterclass

As a special thank-you for purchasing this manual, you'll gain access to an exclusive video course featuring the very best resources on castor oil. Carefully handpicked, this collection of premium videos showcases the most informative and inspiring guides available, offering expert insights and step-by-step demonstrations for beauty, health, and wellness applications.

Whether you're new to castor oil or looking to deepen your knowledge, these top-tier videos provide a powerful visual companion to help you confidently incorporate castor oil's benefits into your life.

Scan the **QR code** below to access this high-value resource

and take your natural self-care journey to the next level!

Or copy and paste the URL:

https://qrco.de/bfcrW3

www.ingramcontent.com/pod-product-compliance
Lightning Source LLC
Chambersburg PA
CBHW081549250726
48653CB00009B/3348